T0266517

The FAMILY FOOD ALLERGY BOOK

The FAMILY FOOD ALLERGY BOOK

A Life Plan You and Your Family Can Live With

Mireille Schwartz

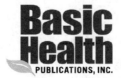

Basic Health
PUBLICATIONS, INC.

This book is not intended as a substitute for medical care of food-allergic individuals, and treatment should not be based solely on its contents. Rather, a practical treatment plan is best developed in a dialogue between each individual and his or her doctor. This book has been written to be an integral part in that diagnosis, conversation, and action plan, so that each food-allergic individual can live a food-allergic life to the fullest.

The publisher does not advocate the use of any particular healthcare protocol but believes the information in this book should be available to the public. The publisher and author are not responsible for any adverse effects or consequences resulting from the use of the suggestions, preparations, or procedures discussed in this book. Should the reader have any questions concerning the appropriateness of any procedures or preparation mentioned, the author and the publisher strongly suggest consulting a professional healthcare advisor.

Excerpts from the Managing Life Threatening Food Allergies in Schools document (pages 53–58) are included by permission of the Massachusetts Department of Elementary and Secondary Education. Inclusion does not constitute endorsement of this book or any other publication. The Managing Life Threatening Food Allergies in Schools document is posted at: www.doe.mass.edu/cnp/allergy.pdf.

Basic Health Publications, Inc.
28812 Top of the World Drive • Laguna Beach, CA 92651
949-715-7327 • www.basichealthpub.com

Library of Congress Cataloging-in-Publication Data

Schwartz, Mireille, 1970-
  The family food allergy book / Mireille Schwartz.
    pages cm
  Includes bibliographical references and index.
  ISBN 978-1-59120-357-5
  1. Food allergy—Diet therapy—Popular works. 2. Food allergy—Diet therapy—
Recipes. I. Title.
  RC588.D53S35 2013
  616.97'3—dc23

                                                      2013036945

Copyright © 2013 by Mireille Schwartz

All rights reserved. No part of this book may be reproduced, stored in a retrieval system, or transmitted by any means, electronic, mechanical, photocopying, recording, or otherwise, without written permission from the author.

Editor: Susan E. Davis
Typesetting/Book design: Gary A. Rosenberg
Cover design: Mike Stromberg

Printed in the United States of America

10   9   8   7   6   5   4   3   2   1

Contents

*This book is dedicated to
Charlotte Jude and Jude Thaddeus,
my Dad,
and Erik
with love and hope.*

Introduction

For the first thirty years of my life, having food allergies was never anything I considered. I had no perspective about my own severe food allergies or food allergies in general. It was, as clichéd as it sounds, something I just didn't think about too much. It was a given: I was severely allergic to fish, I'd always been severely allergic to fish, and there wasn't a darn thing that could be done about it. It didn't define me; it just . . . *was*. Latchkey kids didn't even begin to describe me and my siblings. We were more or less abandoned daily in our home, in conditions which would no doubt be scrutinized and quickly corrected in this day and age. Back then, we were left to try to fend for ourselves all day every day and some nights. It was a disaster fraught with perils, punctuated with kitchen fires, and worse. Despite a strong, unbreakable, and adoring adult relationship I now have with my father and mentor, Dr. Michel Jean-Baptiste, there was nothing in my home to ground me when I was young. I didn't know how to take personal responsibility for my medical condition, and it was clear to me that I wasn't in charge of the bigger picture. Eventually, none too easily or gracefully, I found my way, and that included teaching myself how to manage my severe food allergy and anaphylaxis. Thus, I invented many of the tactics and strategies you'll find in this book. I'm a self-taught food-allergy expert, with a running total of forty years of concrete, independent, hands-on experience.

In this essentially solo operation, I was fortunate to have the help of good, well-meaning friends along the way until one sunny, spectacularly clear June afternoon, in a birthing suite in San Francisco, with sweeping views of the Golden Gate Bridge and an icy ocean dotted with hundreds of sailboats, everything in my life changed. I gave birth and became a mother. And everything I thought I knew, everything I understood, about life changed in an instant. That my daughter, Charlotte Jude, was diagnosed with food allergies at a young age was not a huge surprise to me. But what was surprising was how we managed it so very differently than what I experienced growing up. All things became about teamwork, about partnership, about listening carefully, about planning with the end in mind, about providing excellent and exemplary care to those around me. I was never taught these fundamentals, and I didn't have anything to fall back on or mimic. But, as it turned out, I was a surprisingly quick study. Suddenly, life as I knew it made a lot more sense, and my food-allergy care and treatment made a lot more sense. It dawned on me: I knew a heckuva lot more about an aggressive survival strategy than I thought, and I began to consider food allergy itself as a problem with an actual solution. I began to observe distinct patterns in Charlotte Jude's food allergies and how to minimize and marginalize them—how to make them almost go away. It has been a welcome surprise that the bulk of her food allergies have begun to dissipate as she's grown older, and many of them have disappeared for good.

Unlike many sympathetic guidebooks written by and for parents eager to share their personal experiences coping with food-allergic children, this book is an important resource that for the first time brings together research, organizational guidelines, and definitive, hands-on expertise, making it a unique manual for everyone who knows someone with a food allergy. If you run the numbers, that's just about each and every one of us. *The Family*

Food Allergy Book instructs you about how to figure it all out, what to do, and how to succeed. Allergists as well as medical doctors certainly present a physiological explanation and sensibility, and several of the nation's leading experts have lent their voices to this book. I thank them all in the Acknowledgments at the end of the book, but here I must thank Dr. Scott Sicherer and the Consortium of Food Allergy Research (CoFAR). Their groundbreaking advances, tireless research, and remarkable dedication to a solution have created a momentum unsurpassed in the history of food allergies. However, even as food allergies have developed into a major public health concern, with staggering numbers growing daily, a more well-rounded, complete, personal, human picture of food allergies is needed in the equation as well, for us to not only survive but also thrive. As I learned by becoming mother to Charlotte Jude, you can, even with severe food allergies, lead a daily life full of bravery, gusto, and happiness.

—*Mireille Schwartz*

1

What Is Food Allergy?

I'm not only a parent of a child with food allergies, but I have personal experience with them. A lifetime, actually. I was born severely allergic to fish. In fact, I'm from an atopic family, meaning we are all predisposed to food allergy. My parents as well as my brother and my young daughter suffer from severe food allergy. Between them, my parents are allergic to eggs and chocolate. My brother has a life-threatening reaction to fish so severe he cannot even walk through a seafood department in a grocery market without requiring doctor-prescribed rescue medication. My own allergy is serious enough to warrant carrying rescue medication at all times, and my daughter also carries rescue medications because she has the currently-oh-so-common peanut allergy. My daughter used to be allergic to tree nuts, but luckily she has outgrown some of them.

Three decades ago, when I was a youngster, the outlook on food allergy within the community at large was vastly different than it is now. Food allergy was not publicly recognized as a major public health concern, so education and advocacy about food allergy simply didn't exist. Instead, food allergies were considered vague and very mysterious, and hardly anyone was prepared for allergic reactions to foods. There were no safety guidelines in restau-

5

rants, and many ignorantly thought that severely food-allergic people were "hysterical" or that they simply didn't like a certain food. Auto injectors of epinephrine, used to stave off anaphylaxis (immediate, severe allergic reaction that may be deadly, which will be detailed below), were thought to be primarily used for emergency bee stings. Aside from my pediatrician, who was surprisingly nonchalant about our family's allergies, no one around me seemed to know what to do or how to keep me safe. Babysitters inadvertently fed me the wrong sandwiches; my teachers at elementary school were unable to keep track of who was eating fish around me or—worse—they fed me fish. At holiday time a festive friend of my parents served me a heaping teaspoon of caviar. One year, at a summer fiesta, I ran a tortilla chip through creamy pink dip and savored it before panting and collapsing—it was pureed salmon.

Many food-allergic children secretly think they are going to die. I wondered if I would make it during countless visits to emergency rooms. My lips puffed up and turned blue, my eyes turned brick red as if every capillary had burst at once, and my throat itched and swelled closed. No one thought to have me carry rescue medication or an auto injector, so each and every allergic reaction spiraled out of control. I was forever covered with itchy eczema patches. I developed wheezing. I almost died.

Back then food-allergy management was full of trial and error. But eventually I found my way, teaching myself little steps, which in turn led to big leaps on how to beat this food allergy at its own game, until I learned an innate understanding of the unique set of challenges and successes presented to me all day, every day in order to enjoy a rich quality of life. What was groundbreaking then is commonplace and everyday now. Today, strategy is everything when it comes to food allergy. The actions clearly laid out on these pages are well developed and practiced. They will empower you to manage your family's food allergy with small, simple steps in order to create a life plan you and your family can *live* with.

A SHORT OVERVIEW OF FOOD ALLERGIES

The term "allergy" comes from two Greek words—*allos* for other and *ergon* for action. The term was coined by Viennese pediatrician Baron Clemens von Pirquet in 1906 to mean "altered reactivity." Dr. von Pirquet astutely noticed that patients who had previously received injections of horse serum or smallpox vaccine had speedy, more severe reactions to a second injection. This concept of an immunological reaction was the basis for describing and understanding a hypersensitivity reaction.

Your body is naturally poised to battle invaders and kill viruses, bacteria, and parasites. Normally, it produces antibodies to attack them, performing a valuable function while keeping the body safe. But if you have a reaction to a substance other than what would normally be expected, you are having an allergic reaction. However, in the case of an allergy, substances that are not germs or poisons trigger the same response. People don't expect to get hives when they eat a red tomato, for example. So rather than think of an allergy as a negative reaction, think of it as a valuable immune response in a body that has gone haywire.

The antibodies produced in response to allergens are called IgE antibodies, which cause certain cells to release histamine, a protein that can cause a variety of classic allergy symptoms. In the case of food allergies, these antibodies generally cause one of a cluster of well-understood symptoms. In general, you should strongly suspect an allergy if symptoms begin almost immediately or within minutes after eating, taking medication, or being stung by an insect. However, some allergic reactions can occur after several hours. In rare cases, reactions develop after 24 hours.

At present, food allergy is a growing public health concern in the United States. More than 12 million Americans have food allergies. That's one in twenty-five individuals, or 4 percent of the U.S. population. The incidence of food allergy is highest in young children—one in seventeen among those under age 3. To date, approximately 3 million children in the United States have food allergies. Based on hospital administration sources, the number of emergency room visits due to food-induced anaphylaxis in the United States range from 50,000 to 125,000 a year.

Food allergies can occur at any time during one's life. No one is immune to developing this condition. Adult onset food allergies and intolerances can be particularly confusing because you've become used to a lifetime of eating a certain food, and suddenly without warning you can be in the throes of a reaction.

So how do we retain balance, promote our family's well-being, and keep our sense of humor in the face of this growing epidemic? The prevalence of food allergy appears to be undeniably on the rise, though reasons for this are poorly understood. The immunology and root cause of food allergy remain largely mysterious, and studies are inconclusive about whether food allergies can be prevented. *Currently there is no known cure for food allergies.* When it comes to food allergies and your family's safety, it can certainly feel like there are more questions than answers floating around. The only aspect everyone seems to agree on is: Food allergies can have deadly consequences.

THREE REACTIONS TO FOOD ALLERGIES

There are three main terms that you should know and learn to distinguish between, as each is very different when determining you or your child's diagnosis and treatment: intolerance, hypersensitivity, and anaphylaxis.

Intolerance

The term "food intolerance" means that a food upsets your intestines, yet does not bother any other target organ. Food intolerances are usually due to an enzyme deficiency, such as lactase deficiency, which in turn causes lactose intolerance. Or the intestines may be oversensitive to certain foods, resulting in abdominal discomfort, diarrhea, and bloating. Intolerance is usually a reaction to the protein content of a food, yet you could be intolerant to any part of the food, including sugar and/or additives. So the best defense is a strong offense: Do your best to avoid foods to which you are intolerant in order to avoid discomfort and irritating symptoms.

Hypersensitivity

Here's what goes on in your body when you're hypersensitive to a food. When a suspect protein or allergen develops in your body, it comes into contact with target organs, usually the skin, the lining of the breathing passages, or the intestines. Then the body mobilizes defense troops called antibodies, and a fight breaks out between these allergens and antibodies. Microscopic explosions occur that release chemicals called histamines (hence allergy medicines are called antihistamines) that disturb the integrity of tissues. Blood vessels dilate and produce a rash, fluid leaks out through injured blood vessels causing a runny nose and puffy, watery eyes, or the muscles in the breathing passages go into spasms of wheezing. Even the brain can be bothered by an allergic reaction. A new field of research called "brain allergy" describes the behavioral reactions of the brain when it's bothered by certain foods.

Oral Allergy Syndrome

Oral allergy syndrome (OAS) comes under the heading of hypersensitivity. OAS is perhaps the most common food-related allergy in adults and typically develops in adult hay fever sufferers or people who are allergic to trees and weeds. OAS is not a separate food allergy but rather represents cross-reactivity between distant remnants of tree or weed pollen still found in certain fruits and vegetables. Hence another term for OAS is "pollen-food allergy." The proteins in the pollen and the foods are similar so the antibodies react to both.

Unlike other food allergies, however, an OAS reaction involves itchiness or tingling limited to the mouth, lips, tongue, and throat.

This reaction typically lasts only a few seconds to a few minutes and may even be a one-time occurrence. While at the very least it can be a terrifying experience, it most often resolves naturally on its own. However, if the itchiness does not pass within minutes, an over-the-counter antihistamine such as Benadryl® resolves the reaction. However, in a very small percentage of people, it can progress into something serious. If you are ever in doubt about the severity of an escalating allergic reaction, always call 911.

Often well-cooked, canned, pasteurized, or frozen food offenders cause little to no reaction due to denaturation of the cross-reacting proteins. So if the fruit or vegetable is cooked, in most instances the reaction will not occur because the proteins causing the reaction have been changed. Therefore, OAS is usually limited to eating only uncooked fruits or vegetables. The accompanying table shows common OAS cross-reactions.

ORAL ALLERGY SYNDROME CROSS-REACTIONS

Allergies to specific pollens are associated with OAS reactions to certain foods.

ALLERGY	ASSOCIATED FOOD
Alder pollen	Almonds, apples, celery, cherries, hazelnuts, parsley, peaches, pears, raspberry, strawberry
Birch pollen	Almonds, apples, apricots, avocados, bananas, carrots, celery, cherries, chicory, coriander, fennel, fig, hazelnuts, kiwifruit, nectarines, parsley, parsnips, peaches, pears, peppers, plums, potatoes, prunes, soy, strawberries, wheat
Grass pollen	Fig, melons, oranges, tomatoes
Mugwort pollen	Apples, carrots, celery, coriander, fennel, parsley, peppers, sunflowers
Ragweed pollen	Artichoke, banana, cantaloupe, chamomile or hibiscus tea, cucumber, dandelions, Echinacea, green pepper, honey, honeydew, paprika, sunflower seeds and oil, watermelon, zucchini

Anaphylaxis

Anaphylaxis is a severe, life-threatening allergic reaction that is categorized as a medical emergency. It refers to a collection of symptoms affecting multiple systems in the body that can cause such things as difficulty breathing, changes in heart rate and blood pressure, and loss of consciousness. Anaphylaxis may even trigger severe asthma attacks. These symptoms may include one or more of the following:

Red, watery eyes	Coughing
Runny nose	Wheezing
Flushed, pale skin	Itching of any body part
Change of voice	Swelling of any body part
Bluish (cyanotic) lips and mouth area	Dizziness, change in mental status
Itchy, scratchy lips, tongue, mouth, and/or throat	Fainting or loss of consciousness
Throat tightness or closing	Stomach cramps
Difficulty swallowing	Diarrhea
Difficulty breathing, shortness of breath	Vomiting
	Sense of doom

Two types of anaphylaxis have specific symptoms:

- *Angioedema* includes swelling of the face, throat, genitals, and possibly bowels and arms/legs.

- *Hives* are itchy welts that resemble insect bites and may appear in small groups or over large areas of the skin.

If you or any family member experiences any of these symptoms, call 911 immediately. Seconds count in cases of anaphylaxis, and epinephrine is the only medication that can reverse its symptoms. If you have previously been prescribed an auto injector of epinephrine (commonly referred to as an EpiPen®), administer it at once. If you don't have one on hand, an over-the-counter oral antihistamine such as Benadryl® may help ease symptoms while you wait for medical attention. If allergy symptoms are accompanied by breathing difficulties, wheezing, or other signs of asthma and you have rescue medication handy, for example, an inhaler and spacer prescribed for asthma, use it immediately.

Some food allergies, especially to nuts and shellfish, can be life threatening. The windpipe may go into spasms or the cardiovascular system may go into shock within minutes after a person eats a particular food. If you or your child has had a serious reaction to any food, even severe hives or wheezing, discuss with your doctor or allergist the possibility of keeping an epinephrine auto injector with you at all times for emergencies. This can be a lifesaver if you are not within minutes of an emergency room.

To prepare your family for administering the real medicine, use the practice auto injector, which is packaged with the real one, to learn what to do and how to do it. (There's no needle or medication in the practice pen.) If you or your child accidentally eats a food that has caused a severe reaction, you might want to take the precaution of going immediately to the nearest emergency room and sitting in the waiting room to see what happens. If the reaction is not severe enough to merit emergency treatment, then you can always go home after a short while.

Biphasic Reaction

A biphasic reaction means the allergic person has a second reaction two to six hours after the first reaction, which can be even more symptomatic and dangerous than the first. This often occurs after the first wave of symptoms is under control. Therefore, a period of monitoring for at least six hours in a medical setting— such as the nearest emergency room—is the safest course of action after the first anaphylactic reaction. However, there's no way to predict if or when a person may have a biphasic reaction or a way to prevent one. Nor are there any precautionary steps to take—unfortunately.

THE IMPORANCE OF TESTING

To date, strict avoidance of allergy-causing food is the only way to avoid a reaction. Allergic diseases, such as asthma, allergic rhinitis (commonly known as hay fever), atopic dermatitis (also known as eczema), and food allergy tend to run in families. Frequently, however, no obvious family history of allergy can be found. My family and I survived figuring it out as we went, without the benefit of the widespread knowledge readily available today. When we had sudden, full-blown allergic and anaphylactic reactions at young ages, there was no question what was happening and why. Allergy testing merely confirmed what we already knew and what had been documented through generations. In cases without a genetic inherited tendency, parents and other caretakers are usually the first people to notice their infants' and toddlers' adverse reactions to foods.

If you or a family member has unmistakable food allergy symptoms after eating certain foods, you may be tempted to simply abstain from the food and avoid the time, expense, and hassle of allergy testing. *I do not recommend this course of action and believe this can be a dangerous mistake.* What you think is a fish allergy, for example, may be a reaction to a fairly common parasite. Or you may react after eating French fries, but actually be allergic to fish previously cooked in the same oil. Symptoms you attribute to dairy allergy may be the more treatable condition of lactose intolerance. Even trace amounts of a food allergen can cause a reaction. Most people who've had an allergic reaction to something they ate thought that food was safe for them. Confusing!

As a parent, I have never underestimated the power of my own gut instincts around food allergy. If you have a hunch, a funny feeling, or a worry, do not hesitate to check it out. Children as

WHAT CHILDREN MIGHT SAY TO DESCRIBE THEIR ALLERGIC REACTION

"My throat/tongue/lips are itchy."

"My throat hurts/is burning."

"There's something poking in my mouth/throat."

"My mouth/tongue/throat feels funny."

Is It a Food Allergy Reaction or Not?

When a possible food allergy is being evaluated and diagnosed, the first step is to determine if the symptoms align with the description of a true immune response to a certain food or foods. Sometimes people have adverse reactions to foods that are not food allergies. For example, food poisoning will typically result in severe gastrointestinal symptoms and can sometimes even closely mimic an allergic reaction with hives, rash, itchy mouth, and vomiting. Working closely with your doctor when diagnosing a food allergy is key, and initial skin prick and blood tests are excellent methods to ensure actual evidence of a potential food allergy.

young as a few months old can begin giving telltale, subtle signs only a parent or caregiver might notice. Colicky baby? Rashes? Stomach upset? All could be the beginning signs of food allergy, as a repetitive pattern begins to form. If you are a parent, ask yourself: Does my child always have this sort of diaper rash after he or she has eaten eggs? If you begin to notice regular, specific physiological trends after a certain food group is consumed, you may well be onto something. Jot it down and talk to your doctor or pediatrician as soon as possible to share your observations. Although it can be frightening to ask these questions, just remember: It's easier to put out a small stovetop fire than it is after everything is engulfed in flames.

If you observe that your child has developed such symptoms as rash, hives, swelling, vomiting, or coughing and wheezing, write down all the foods and ingredient lists of suspect foods the child ate within 24 hours prior to the reaction while everything is still fresh in your mind. If you ate at a relative's home or in a restaurant, ask your host or the restaurant personnel who cooked the offending food for the specific items included in the dish. Try to assess whether your child has eaten these foods regularly or rarely in the past. Also consider sources of cross-contamination: What was the food in contact with prior to entering the child's mouth? Make sure you list the dates, times, and locations where potential attacks occurred.

Once you think you have identified a particular food as a potential allergen, it is essential that the child strictly avoid eating any of the food until a medical allergy evaluation is completed by an allergist, and a clear and definitive diagnosis is made. In the meantime, that same day, contact your child's primary care provider and discuss the need for an epinephrine auto injector (brands are EpiPen® or Twinject®). The next step is making an appointment for an allergy evaluation with the allergist recommended by your primary care physician.

The Allergy Evaluation

The evaluation begins with a thorough history of the child, including information about all reactions that have occurred when your child has consumed certain foods. Then the allergist will assess your child's personal and family history of allergies and perform a physical examination looking for signs of allergic disease. It is important to realize that often the history is far more important than the examination, and it's not necessary for the allergist to see your child while in the midst of an acute reaction. When the history and exam are completed, it's time to discuss testing recommendations and develop a personalized action plan for your child. Typically, the skin and blood tests described below will be ordered swiftly for your child, and you will be given written instructions and extensive education regarding food avoidance, which is essential for your child's safety. There are also community support groups that can help you assess the day-to-day needs for your child as you begin to implement the necessary changes in your life and household. Your allergist will have this information readily available.

Food allergy evaluations are really a partnership, and much more is involved in the diagnosis of a true food allergy than doing a quick and easy skin or blood test. Understanding the types of reactions the child has to certain foods, the timing of eating the food in relationship to these reactions, the child's personal history, and the family history—all these elements are critical to a comprehensive food allergy evaluation. The best results occur when the parents, child, and healthcare provider work together, each sharing his or her area of knowledge to help with the diagnosis and management of a food allergy. You may come to depend on your allergist as a comrade or even a friend.

Your allergist can confirm a food-allergy diagnosis by performing one or both of the following standard laboratory tests.

Skin Test

For a skin or prick test, the child is pricked with a series of needles that contain extracts of allergic triggers. The allergist then looks for strong reactions like welts or red bumps to determine if the patient has allergies. While a skin test is helpful in uncovering food allergies, it does have a high incidence of false positives, meaning the test shows the child is allergic to a food when he or she really isn't. A negative skin test is a much more reliable indication that the child is unlikely to be allergic to that food.

Blood Test

For an allergy blood test, called a RAST (Radio-Allergo-Sorbent Test), a sample of the patient's blood is sent to a laboratory for analysis, where antibodies in the blood are tested on certain food allergens. The suspected allergen is bound to an insoluble material, and drops of the patient's blood are added. If the blood serum contains antibodies to the allergen, then those antibodies will bind to the allergen. (This test is also known as the ImmunoCAP Specific IgE blood test because it provides IgE levels, which indicate allergy.) The allergist carefully examines these test results to determine if the patient has allergies.

A positive blood test is a reliable indicator that you or your child is likely to be allergic to that food. If a certain food, say, peanuts, shows up positive on a RAST, that means your child is more likely than not to be allergic to peanuts. This is my preferred method of testing for food allergy, especially when a patient has such a high sensitivity level to suspected allergens that any administration of those allergens directly into the skin could result in potentially serious side effects.

2

The Big 8 Allergy-Causing Foods

E ight foods—I refer to them as the "Big 8"—account for 90 percent of all food-allergic reactions in the United States: milk, eggs, peanuts, tree nuts (including almonds, cashews, pecans, pistachios, and walnuts), wheat, soy, fish, and shellfish. The following list provides basic information about each food and obvious and hidden sources of the food. Note that special care is needed when determining hidden sources of allergy-causing foods, especially when purchasing prepared products and eating in restaurants or in other people's homes. Because reading all the ingredients listed in labels is so important, that will be covered in detail in Chapter 3, Changing Your Lifestyle.

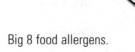

Big 8 food allergens.

1. MILK

A milk allergy is an adverse immune reaction to one or more elements of milk from any animal, most commonly alpha S1-casein, a protein in cow's milk. According to the National Center for Health Statistics, approximately 2.5 percent of U.S. children younger than 3 years of age are allergic to milk. Nearly all infants who develop an allergy to milk do so in the first year of life, and most children who have milk allergy will outgrow it in the first few years of life. However, a 2007 study published in the November issue of the *Journal of Allergy and Clinical Immunology* has shown that milk allergy may persist longer in life than previously thought. According to a study of 800 children with milk allergy, only 19 percent had outgrown their allergy by age 4, and only 79 percent had outgrown it by age 16.[1]

Milk is sometimes referred to as casein, caseinate, sodium caseinate, and lactose. Also referred to as hydrolysates (casein, milk protein, protein, whey, whey protein) lactalbumin, lactalbumin phosphate, lactoglobulin, and lactulose. In addition, the letter D on the front label of a product indicates the product may contain cow's milk protein.

Milk is found in the following foods.

- Butter
- Cheese
- Chowders
- Cottage cheese
- Cream
- Curds
- Custards or puddings
- Deli meats and luncheon meats, including sausages and hot dogs
- Half & half
- Ice cream and sherbet
- Margarine
- Mashed potatoes and instant mashed potatoes
- Sheep and goat milk and cheese
- Sour cream
- Yogurt

Hidden milk food sources.

- Artificial butter flavor

- Baby formulas

- Canned tuna fish contains casein

- Caramel color and caramel flavoring

- Deli meat slicers often used for both meat and cheese products

- Many nondairy products contain casein so check labels carefully

2. EGGS

Egg allergy is a hypersensitivity to dietary substances made with the yolk and/or whites of eggs, which causes an overreaction of the immune system. Someone who has an allergic reaction to the egg yolk may be able to easily tolerate egg whites, and vice versa. Many egg-allergic individuals, however, are allergic to proteins in both the egg yolk and the egg white. Egg allergy is estimated to affect approximately 1.5 percent of young children, and it's one of the most likely allergies to be outgrown over time.

Eggs are found in the following food sources.

- Albumin

- Battered fish, battered poultry, and battered meat

- Cake, muffins, cream pies, cream puffs, and soufflés

- Creamed soups

- Custards or puddings

- Eggnog

- French toast

- Frosting, custards, marshmallows, and meringue

- Hollandaise sauce

- Ice cream

- Mayonnaise

- Some egg substitutes contain egg whites

- Tartar sauce

- Waffles

Hidden egg food sources.

- Dry pastas that are boxed and commercial are usually egg-free, but most are processed on equipment that is also used for egg-containing products.

- Egg white glaze is sometimes used on pretzels before they are dipped in salt and may also be found on shiny baked goods and pastries.

- Foam topping is sometimes used on specialty coffee drinks and some bar drinks, for example, Pisco.

3. PEANUTS

Peanut allergy is a reaction to dietary substances from peanuts causing an overreaction of the immune system. The Asthma and Allergy Foundation of America estimates that peanut allergy is one of the most common causes of food-related death. Peanut allergies are on the rise in children in the United States, but currently there is no confirmed medical treatment to prevent or cure the allergic reaction to peanuts. If you are allergic to peanuts, you may develop allergies to tree nuts, and vice versa.

Peanuts are found in the following food sources.

- Baked goods, for example, scones, muffins, and breads

- Desserts, for example, ice creams, brownies, and cookies

- Energy bars and candies

- Glazes and marinades

- Nougat

- Peanut butter

- Peanut oil

- Sauces, for example, satay sauce for chicken, pesto, and mole

- Soups

Hidden peanut food sources.

- Alternative nut butters; for example, some sunflower seed and soy butters are made on equipment shared with peanuts; always read labels and/or contact the manufacturer

- Asian, Thai, and Mexican dishes

- Chili

- Chocolates

- Compost (manufactured for lawns or gardens) often contains peanut shells or hulls

- Egg rolls and spring rolls

- Fried foods; always ask if peanut oil is used

- Orange juice: Only Minute Maid Heart Wise® orange juice contains plant sterols derived from peanut oil

- Pet foods

- Pizzas, especially gourmet

- Vegetarian and meat-substitute products

4. TREE NUTS

Tree nut allergy is a hypersensitivity to dietary substances in tree nuts, which causes an overreaction of the immune system. Tree nuts include almonds, Brazil nuts, cashews, chestnuts, filberts/hazelnuts, macadamia nuts, pecans, pine nuts/pignolia nuts, pistachios, hickory nuts, and walnuts. Individuals with tree nut allergies are seldom allergic to just one type of nut. An estimated 1.8 million Americans have an allergy to tree nuts. Allergic reactions to tree nuts are the second leading cause of fatal and near-fatal reactions to foods. Some people who are allergic to peanuts are also allergic to tree nuts, and vice versa.

Tree nuts are found in the following food sources.

- Almonds, including marzipan and amaretto (distillated from kernels)
- Brazil nuts
- Cashews
- Chestnuts
- Filberts/hazelnuts
- Hickory nuts
- Macadamia nuts
- Nut butter, nut paste, and nut extract
- Pecans
- Pine nuts
- Pistachio nuts
- Walnuts

Hidden tree nut food sources.

- Barbecue sauce
- Breading for chicken and meats
- Deli meats; for example, mortadella contains pistachio nuts
- Gluten-free flours and gluten-free pancake and bake mixes
- Honey
- Pancakes
- Pastas
- Piecrusts and cake
- Salads and salad dressings
- Vegetarian and meat-substitute products

5. WHEAT

Wheat allergy is a hypersensitivity to dietary substances from wheat proteins causing an overreaction of the immune system. More than twenty different potential wheat allergens have been identified. Wheat allergy is sometimes confused with Celiac disease, which is a digestive disorder that creates an adverse reaction to gluten. Individuals with Celiac disease must avoid gluten, found in wheat, rye, barley, and sometimes oats. Celiac disease and gluten sensitivity are not an allergic reaction to wheat.

CELIAC DISEASE VERSUS WHEAT ALLERGY

Celiac disease and wheat allergies share wheat as the culprit, but the two conditions differ considerably. Celiac disease is a genetic auto-immune disease; it causes the body to produce antibodies that attack the villi in the small intestine when the affected person consumes gluten, which is a protein in wheat. Symptoms are typically gastrointestinal in nature and include chronic diarrhea and constipation, abdominal bloating, and pain. Celiac disease may begin at any age, and the average length of time for a symptomatic person to be diagnosed is 4 years. People with a wheat allergy can grow out of it. Because Celiac disease is a genetic disorder, people have the condition for life.

Wheat is found in the following food sources.

- Beer (some beers contain wheat)
- Bread and bread crumbs
- Bulgur
- Cereal extract, bran, and wheat germ
- Couscous
- Cracker meal
- Durum
- Farina
- Flour: all-purpose flour, enriched flour, and high-protein flour
- "Natural" flavoring
- Pasta
- Semolina wheat
- Soy sauce
- Starch
- Vegetable gum

Hidden wheat food sources.

- Alcohol: bourbon, gin, scotch, whiskey, and some wines
- Baked beans
- Communion wafers
- Hot dogs
- Ice cream
- Instant mashed potatoes
- Marinara sauce

- Play Doh
- Potato chips
- Rice cakes

6. SOY

Soy protein allergy is a hypersensitivity to dietary substances from soy causing an overreaction of the immune system. (Soy is sometimes referred to as lecithin.) Soy allergies usually appear during childhood, but adult-onset soy allergies are possible as well. Soy is widely used in processed food and in a multitude of products, for example, chewing gums and peanut butter.

Soy is found in the following food sources.

- Canned tuna
- Edamame
- Infant formula
- Lecithin or soy lecithin
- Miso
- Monosodium glutamate (MSG)
- Soy flour
- Soy grits
- Soy meal
- Soy milk
- Soy oil
- Soy sauce
- Tamari and tamari sauce
- Tempeh
- Tofu
- Vegetable oil
- Vitamin E

Hidden soy food sources.

- Bouillon cubes (vegetable, chicken, beef, and so on)
- Caramel coloring
- Cereal
- Chewing gum
- Chicken broth, canned
- Crackers
- Fast-food restaurant hamburger meat and hamburger buns
- Peanut butter
- Sauces
- Soups

HIDDEN SOY IN EVERYDAY ITEMS

There are many other sources of soy in day-to-day life: adhesives, blankets, body lotions and creams, dog foods, enamel paints, fabric finishes and some fabrics, fertilizers, flooring materials, lubricants, nitroglycerine medication, paper, printer inks, and even some shampoos and soaps.

---

7. FISH

Fish allergy is a hypersensitivity to dietary substances in fish that cause an overreaction of the immune system. According to a recent Mt. Sinai Hospital study, 2.8 percent of adult Americans are allergic to fish and shellfish.[2]

The primary allergen in fish is called parvalbumin. According to the National Center for Health Statistics, 40 percent of people with a fish allergy experience their first allergic reaction as an adult. Over 50 percent of fish-allergy sufferers are allergic to more than one type of fish. Allergic reactions may result when the susceptible person is not even consuming the allergenic substance, but he or she is exposed to vapors from fish being cooked or even fish preparation or handling in a kitchen or restaurant.

Fish is found in the following food sources.

- Anchovies
- Artificial crabmeat or imitation crabmeat
- Bouillabaisse and fish stocks and soups
- Caviar (fish eggs)
- Ceviche
- Fish oil and dietary supplement fish oil capsules
- Fish sticks
- Flounder
- Grouper
- Halibut

- Orange juice fortified with calcium supplement

- Salad dressing, for example, Caesar dressing (containing anchovies) or Menhaden oil dressing

- Salmon

- Sardines

- Seafood flavoring

- Snapper

- Sole

- Tilapia

- Tuna

- Worcestershire sauce (containing anchovies) and barbecue sauces that contain Worcestershire sauce

Hidden fish food sources.

- Asian foods that contain fish oils, fish powders and flakes, fish sauces

- Beer: Some nut brown or English brown ales contain fish

- Burgers and steaks in restaurants are sometimes accompanied with anchovy powder or anchovy barbecue sauce for enhanced flavor

- Cat foods

- Caesar salad dressings may contain anchovy

- Glucosamine, for example, Osteo Bi-Flex arthritis supplement

- Omega-3 oil and Omega-6 oil; for example, Jif Omega-3 peanut butter contains anchovy oil, sardine oil, and tilapia

- Organic plant foods

8. SHELLFISH

Shellfish allergy is a hypersensitivity to dietary substances from shellfish causing an overreaction of the immune system. An esti-mated 7 million Americans are allergic to seafood, including fish and shellfish. There are several types of shellfish, and each kind contains different allergy-causing proteins. *Crustaceans* include crabs, lobster, crayfish, shrimp, and prawn. *Mollusks* include bivalves, such as clams, mussels, oysters, and scallops; gastropods, such as limpets, periwinkles, snails (escargot), and abalone; and cephalopods, such as squid, cuttlefish, and octopus. Shrimp, crab, and lobster cause most shellfish allergies.

When shellfish is cooked, its proteins become airborne, and the inhalation of the cooking vapors or steam in a kitchen or restaurant may cause a severe allergic reaction. Other shellfish allergic reactions may occur from simply handling shellfish.

Shellfish is found in the following food sources.

- Abalone
- Bouillabaisse and fish stocks and soups
- Clams and mussels
- Cockles
- Crustaceans, for example, shrimp, crab, lobster, and crawfish
- Octopus
- Oysters
- Sea urchins
- Seafood flavoring
- Snails or escargot
- Squid

Hidden shellfish food sources.

- Asian foods may contain shellfish sauces and shellfish powders and flakes
- Coral calcium supplements and additives
- Glucosamine, for example, Osteo Bi-Flex arthritis supplement
- Omega-3 oil and Omega-6 oil used in a wide variety of prepared foods, including margarine
- Vitamin dietary supplements

ALLERGENS IN NOT-FOOD SUBSTANCES

Be certain to carefully check soaps, lotions, cosmetics, and toiletries for potentially allergenic ingredients that might end up on your hands or your mouth. Other possible sources of allergens include:

Adhesives: Many lick-and-stick adhesive stamps and envelopes contain wheat. Some older stationery envelopes contain fish.

Body lotions: Many contain tree nut oils, peanut oil, and fish oils. Some also contain extracts of wheat.

Makeup: Lipsticks and creamy makeup may include wheat and tree nut oils.

Medications: Always check the active and inactive ingredients list in over-the-counter medications as some may contain wheat, soy, and milk.

Paints: Some contain food ingredients so always check with the manufacturer.

Pet foods: Many contain wheat, milk, peanut, and egg. Bird seeds may also contain many peanut and tree nut products.

Play Doh: Check to see if it contains wheat.

Shampoos and conditioners: Some may contain wheat or extracts of wheat, almond, and tree nut oils, soy, and even fish oils.

Vitamins and supplements: Always check the ingredients list as many contain wheat, soy, milk, peanuts, tree nuts, and fish products.

3

Changing Your Lifestyle

If a skin test and a blood test agree, then it's confirmed: You or your family member has a food allergy. That means you must change your lifestyle to stay safe and sane!

Once back home, as soon as you can, clear out every item you or your family member can't eat from your pantry, refrigerator, and freezer. It's also a good idea to thoroughly clean and sanitize your pantry, refrigerator, freezer, oven, stove top, cooking utensils, and cookware—even if that means replacing certain cooking utensils and cookware or having two sets of things for different kinds of preparations. Why? Keeping unsafe items out of your food preparation and storage areas—or segregating them in some way—will reduce opportunities for *cross-contamination*. When preparing and serving food, it is critical to make sure that food preparation and serving utensils are not exposed to allergens and then used when preparing or serving other foods. Food production areas in the kitchen should be cleaned before, during, and after food preparation. Some examples of cross-contamination are:

- Lifting peanut butter cookies with a spatula and then using it to lift sugar cookies.

- Using a knife to make peanut butter sandwiches, wiping the knife with a damp cloth, and then using the knife to spread mustard on a cheese sandwich for a peanut-allergic child.

Food allergies are a proven source of stress, and the early adjustment period can be extremely difficult. Remember that what might seem like a huge amount of work in the beginning quickly becomes familiar, routine, and easy, though remaining vigilant is key.

TWO-STEP PROCESS TO STAY HEALTHY

Since there is no known cure for food allergies, avoidance is the most effective means of surviving successfully with your allergy. So the next step is to identify the triggers and teach yourself or your loved one how to reduce exposure to them. You'd be surprised how quickly you will be able to adapt to you or your family member's food allergy. Day by day it will become much easier to manage. You will learn how to worry less and enjoy life while staying attentive at the same time.

As a young child living with a food allergy and after repeated exposures to fish—both ingested and inhaled—that led to countless terrifying allergic reactions, I became highly adaptable in order to stay alive. I didn't want to die from a violent reaction, and I feared I would unless I figured out a way to not only avoid my allergen but also live life "outside a bubble." I didn't want to dread dining out, have anxiety around dating and intimacy, and forego a lifetime of incredible, enriching adventures with family, friends, and loved ones. So I taught myself tricks and tactics to work around fish in every conceivable situation. With multiple decades of trial and error, practice, and experience, I have developed a lifelong, well-tested, daily prophylactic action strategy for survival, plus an emergency rescue plan for myself. With forethought and some practice this can also work wonders for you and your family.

Step 1: The Life Cycle of Your Meals

Success in managing food allergies depends on savvy allergen-avoidance techniques. Consistently reading ingredient labels of all foods is the first and major part of Step 1.

If a packaged product doesn't have a label, then you categorically should not buy or eat that food. You can't afford to risk it. Whenever you have doubts, always contact the manufacturer for more information. Many food manufacturers have consumer response departments that provide information about their products.

The Food and Drug Administration created the Food Allergen Labeling and Consumer Protection Act (FALCPA) of 2004. This ensures that all Big 8 allergens are accurately labeled on everything from frozen dinners to candy bars to even prewashed and bagged salads. Ingredient lists must include the Big 8 in plain language, and allergenic ingredients must be listed even if they are only present in trace amounts, including as colors, flavors, and/or in spice blends. The specific type of tree nut and specific type of fish and shellfish must be specified, for example, walnut or almond and cod, crab, or shrimp.

To date, however, FALCPA does not require declaration of allergenic ingredients introduced through cross-contamination. That occurs when a trace amount of an allergen is unintentionally incorporated into another food, usually when machines or equipment in food-producing factories are not cleaned thoroughly between different operations. This labeling step is immensely helpful in understanding the entire life cycle of any food product, which starts with the production of all raw materials and assesses every step of the food-making process through labeling and packaging to make sure none of the Big 8 sneaks in.

Fortunately, many manufacturers have voluntarily adopted allergen advisory labels that address cross-contamination during the manufacturing process. Most of them make every effort to eliminate or reduce the risk of the unintentional presence of allergens in factories. And they work diligently to identify the critical points where allergens could be introduced during manufacturing and cleaning equipment or even where products could be incorrectly labeled. The end result is a product with an informational label such as "Made on equipment shared with eggs" or "May contain peanuts."

To prevent accidental exposure, it is vital to read all labels scrupulously on every prepared food item before you purchase it. You need to become a knowledgeable interpreter of ingredient statements. For instance, a phrase like "Plant sterols" could also mean peanut, and even "Spices" might include an allergen. If you have any questions, any at all, about a product ingredient, call the consumer hotline number listed on the food label. Be certain to have the package in hand so the hotline operator can work with you to reference the bar code identification number on the product. This will enable the operator to cross-reference your package with exact, up-to-date precision regarding where, when, and how the product was prepared. Be specific. For example, ask, "Does your product include peanuts? Is there a risk of cross-contamination with peanuts in your food manufacturing process?" Manufacturers are accustomed to answering such questions.

It's important to understand that recipes of packaged products sometimes change, so you should read a label each and every time you consider buying a product—even if it is a product with which you are familiar. Luckily, some foods are prepared in a dedicated facility, meaning the food is produced in a facility that is free from a specific allergen or allergens. Dedicated facilities offer the highest level of protection because their products are completely safe from cross-contamination.

Once you begin to think about all your meals—every single one—and all the foods your child or you can and cannot eat as part of your entire "life cycle," you'll soon be able to have a conversation about your allergy or your child's allergy with parents at your child's school prior to a group celebration, with friends before you attend their dinner parties, with chefs at local restaurants, even with a catering company before a wedding. (How to have such conversations is spelled out in Chapter 4, Coping with the Diagnosis.) This comprehensive, sensible strategy will not only help your child or you avoid the allergen but also help protect everyone from the chance of dangerous cross-contamination while eating what should be safe foods.

HOW TO READ LABELS
TO AVOID FOOD ALLERGENS

The following section on reading labels is reprinted with permission from the Consortium of Food Allergy Research (CoFAR).

U.S. law requires that food labels clearly identify the source of ingredients derived from these eight major food allergens:

Milk   **Soybean (Soya)**   **Wheat**

Egg   **Peanut**

Tree nut—the specific tree nut must be identified.

Fish—the specific fish species must be identified.

Crustacean shellfish—the specific species must be identified (e.g., shrimp, lobster, crab).*

*Mollusks (e.g., clams, oysters, scallops) are not considered "major allergens" under US law and therefore are not necessarily identified on labels.

Read the Entire Label (not just the list of ingredients because allergen statements may appear elsewhere) each and every time you purchase an item.

Ingredients: Read the entire ingredient list, including any "contains" or advisory statements and look specifically for those ingredients you need to avoid.

The law only applies to the eight foods/food groups that are considered the "major allergens." If you are allergic to other foods (such as seeds, garlic or any others), you will need to call the manufacturer to know if ingredients labeled with non-specific terms such as "spice" or "natural flavoring" contain a food you are avoiding.

Unintentional ingredients and "May Contain" advisory statements: The unintentional presence of ingredients due to contamination or cross contact in processing is not required to be listed on the product label.

Some manufacturers choose to use advisory labeling to address the issue of unintentional ingredients. Look for advisory labeling such as "may contain [allergen]" or "produced in a facility that also produces [allergen]."

Beware: The words used may not reflect risk (for example, "in a facility" may not be safer than "may contain"). Avoid any product that contains an advisory statement for your allergen, regardless of the type of advisory statement used.

As advisory labeling is voluntary, the absence of an advisory statement does not necessarily mean there is no risk of cross contact with an allergen.

A Sample Chicken Soup Label with an Advisory Statement:

The ingredient list in the sample chicken soup label includes milk. This product label also carries an advisory statement—although the ingredient list does not indicate the presence of egg or wheat, the advisory statement indicates that there is a risk of cross contact with egg or wheat; therefore, this product would not be considered safe for those with milk, egg, or wheat allergy:

Nutrition Facts	Amount/serving	%DV*	Amount/serving	%DV*
Serv. Size 1 cup (249g)	**Total Fat** 12g	**18%**	**Sodium** 940mg	**39%**
Servings About 2	Sat. Fat 6g	**30%**	**Total Carb.** 24g	**8%**
Calories 250	Polyunsat. Fat 1.5g		Dietary Fiber 1g	**4%**
Fat Cal. 110	Monounsat. Fat 2.5g		Sugars 1g	
*Percent Daily Values (DV) are based on a 2,000 calorie diet.	**Cholest.** 60mg	**20%**	**Protein** 10g	**20%**
	Vitamin A 0% • VitaminC 0% • Calcium 6% • Iron 8%			

Ingredients: WATER, CHICKEN, RICE, MODIFIED CORN STARCH, CREAM (MILK), POTATO, CARROT, ONION, SPICES, SALT. **MAY CONTAIN EGG AND WHEAT**

Kosher Pareve:

Although a product labeled OU Pareve or Kosher Pareve should not contain milk ingredients, the pareve certification is not a guarantee that the product is safe for those allergic to milk. Always read the label and call the manufacturer before assuming a product is safe.

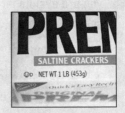

Kosher Dairy:

Ingredients: ENRICHED FLOUR (WHEAT FLOUR, NIACIN, REDUCED IRON, THIAMINE MONONITRATE [VITAMIN B1], RIBOFLAVIN [VITAMIN B2], FOLIC ACID), SOYBEAN OIL, SALT, PARTIALLY HYDROGENATED COTTONSEED OIL, BAKING SODA, MALTED BARLEY FLOUR, CALCIUM CARBONATE (SOURCE OF CALCIUM), YEAST.

The D following the U indicates that this product is considered a dairy food by kosher law and the product either contains a dairy ingredient., or the product does not contain a dairy ingredient but was made on equipment that also makes other products with dairy ingredients. This cracker is considered kosher dairy due to the potential for milk contamination in the product. This product and other Kosher Dairy products are not considered safe for those with milk allergy.

More Label Reading Tips

Read the label each time: Ingredients change! Different brands of a product, such as bread, may have different ingredients.

Labeling laws DO NOT cover medications or cosmetics that could have food ingredients.

You may need to contact the manufacturer for more information about a product:

• To ask the manufacturer about cross contact risk.

- To find out if ambiguous terms (e.g., "spices") could be the allergen you are avoiding if your allergen is not part of the labeling laws (e.g., sesame, garlic, etc. are not required to be on the label).

  ○ Manufacturers may be reluctant to reveal "secret ingredients."

  ○ Ask specific questions such as: "My child is allergic to sesame; do the 'spices' contain sesame?" instead of asking "What spices are used?"

© Consortium of Food Allergy Research NIAID Grant U19 AI 066738. The Consortium of Food Allergy Research (CoFAR) was established in July 2005 by the National Institute of Allergy and Infectious Diseases (NIAID) to conduct both observational and clinical studies to answer questions related to food allergies.

STEP 2: Your Food-Allergy Grab-n-Go Bag

Strict avoidance of an allergy-causing food, along with awareness and comprehension of the life cycle of your meals, is your best daily strategy. Nonetheless, it's essential to carry a food-allergy emergency medical bag at all times. It should contain 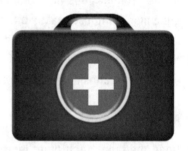 several doses of up-to-date antihistamines such as Bendaryl® in an easy-to-swallow form and an inhaler and spacer if you have asthma, and it's recommended that you carry two epinephrine auto injectors in case a second dose is necessary. The bag should be small enough to fit into a fanny pack or a backpack compartment. My small grab-n-go is red so it's easy to identify.

Contents of Your Food-Allergy Grab-n-Go Bag

- Two epinephrine auto injectors, as prescribed by your doctor.

- Antihistamine in easy-to-swallow form: melt-away strip or liquid.

- Asthma inhaler and pacer, if suggested by your doctor.

- Emergency contact information with names and telephone numbers of your doctor and people you want contacted in case of an emergency.

As you become accustomed to toting your medicine around with you, it's important to avoid exposing your grab-n-go bag to extreme heat or cold. For example, a seemingly good but unacceptable place to keep your medication is in your car's glove compartment. After all, you're always in your car, right? Wrong. You must *never* store your medical bag in the glove compartment of your vehicle as temperatures can soar to over 100°F (38°C) in the interior and epinephrine breaks down in heat. Ideally, your auto injector should be stored at 77°F (25°C). However, the range of 59°–86°F (15°–30°C) is permitted. These temperature fluctuations are fine when storing the auto injector, as well as when you carry the bag during the course of a day. But if the medication is exposed to temperatures outside this range, the product will be compromised. Even under perfect conditions, auto injectors have a relatively short shelf life, though proper storage can help extend it a little. The product starts to visibly deteriorate at or around the expiration date. When I get new auto injectors from the pharmacy, I mark the expiration date on my calendar, so I'm sure to see it coming up and have plenty of advance notice of when it's time to replace the medication.

Because epinephrine auto injectors are packaged with practice injectors, which don't contain needles or any medication, you can practice with the decoy injector on yourself, with friends and family, and with appropriate staff at your child's school. Similar to cardiopulmonary resuscitation (CPR) training, the more you practice the better equipped you'll be in an actual emergency when every second counts. You can't really practice too much. Fortu-

nately, the lifesaving steps of administering the auto injector will
soon become second nature. I like to think: I practice this often
with my community at large in the hope of never having to use
it, so I'm 100 percent certain to be prepared.

Part of living with food allergy is recognizing that epinephrine
is the first line of defense for treating life-threatening allergic reactions. If you or your child begins to feel aggressive symptoms, all
efforts should be directed toward the immediate use of an auto
injector. Do not attempt to sneak off to a restroom for privacy to
administer your meds. Instead, tell someone nearby exactly what
is happening, so they can aid you, stay by your side, and call 911
if necessary. It can take a deceptively short amount of time to succumb to an allergic reaction and become incapacitated, and no
two allergic reactions are exactly alike.

Remember, a person can't tell how severe his or her next food-
allergy reaction will be based on the severity of previous reactions.
So while it's important not to panic, it's equally important to

AUTO INJECTOR DISPOSAL: HOW TO DO IT SAFELY

How to use, care for, and store an auto injector quickly becomes common knowledge among those who require one. However, disposing of
a needle many inches long chock full of a foreign agent can prove tax-
ing and potentially nerve wracking. Many who have experienced anaphylaxis have a small collection of expired or faulty auto injectors at
home without any idea of how or where to correctly dispose of them.
Here are some options—and preparations you can make—when you
need to dispose of an auto injector.

After you use it, place the auto injector in the plastic case it came
in. Carefully avoid the exposed needle at the head of the injector while
doing that, and screw the large green lid on as tightly as possible. You

may want to do this over a napkin or paper towel in case any solution left in the injector drips out of the syringe.

Call the following professionals to confirm if they will assist you in properly disposing of an auto injector. Healthcare professionals vary greatly in the services they provide, so take the time to pick up the phone before assuming any of the following will accept your injector and before you need to dispose of one.

- **Your pharmacist** disposes of his or her own stock of expired auto injectors and will often take other people's as well. They also know their customers—perhaps they even filled your prescription—and you will not be suspect when you walk in with a tube full of adrenaline. Bonus for you: At the same time you can get a new auto injector prescription filled to replace the one you're throwing away and save yourself a trip.

- **Your doctor's office** will have a special "sharps" disposal and sometimes will take auto injectors as well.

- **Your local hospital, its emergency room, or the allergy clinic in your local hospital** may all accept an auto injector for disposal, given that they will be disposing of their own used sharps and needles daily.

- **Medical labs**, especially those where blood is drawn with needles or blood work is routinely processed, will sometimes take auto injector for disposal. Be sure to ask if the facility charges a fee for disposing of your auto injector. Many do. If so, it's well worth an extra couple of minutes to call the next professional on the list to get the service for free.

- **Household garbage** can be used as a last resort if an injector has been used, certain precautions are observed, and all other options fail. *Use extreme care to ensure that the injector is completely secure in its plastic case. Place the injector directly into a garbage can that cannot under any circumstances be accessed by a child.*

optimize every second to manage your health crisis quickly and efficiently. When in doubt, always administer the medication and always call 911 or ask whoever is with you to do so. It helps to stay focused, and remember that you can get through this. Breathe as deeply and regularly as you can and stay as alert as possible. Be certain to describe any rapid changes to those around you. By now you've practiced many times, and *you know what to do to help with your own or your family member's medical condition.* Emergency personnel will arrive speedily and can always evaluate the situation appropriately and then depart once the allergic reaction has stabilized and subsided.

Knowing where the closest hospital is to your home, your workplace, your child's school, or your usual travel routes is essential. It's good to practice driving these routes prior to an emergency, so you know where the emergency loading zones are. This will help you stay alert during a situation that feels like it's rapidly spinning out of control. Even if you only plan to drive a short distance, this is a key time not to be alone. You will be amazed at how helpful a friend or even a Good Samaritan can be once you quickly and calmly alert them to the situation. Keep in mind: Since exposure to allergy-causing foods is typically accidental, being able to treat the reaction immediately with the epinephrine auto injector in your grab-n-go bag is paramount. You should practice, practice, practice and always be prepared to recognize and treat an allergic reaction as quickly as you possibly can.

4

Coping with the Diagnosis

At first it can feel like a diagnosis of food allergies is insurmountable and your family's life will be dramatically altered and restricted. This book is dedicated to helping you develop lifesaving habits and become an expert at dealing with food allergies. You will find that day-to-day family life can still be normal and festive once you learn what steps are involved in protecting your family member from a certain food or foods. Now that you're aware of that two-step process detailed in the last chapter, let's take a look at the most immediate emotional and social issues confronting families who cope with food allergies.

WILL MY CHILD OUTGROW A FOOD ALLERGY?

The most common question parents of food-allergic children ask is: How likely is it that my child will outgrow his or her food allergy? The answer to that question differs for various foods. Most children allergic to cow's milk, egg, soy, and wheat will outgrow this allergy between the ages of 3 and 16 years. In contrast, allergies to peanuts, tree nuts, fish, and shellfish are generally lifelong allergies. However, studies have shown that approximately 20 percent of children may outgrow their allergy to peanuts, while about 10 percent outgrow their allergy to tree nuts.

Your allergist can use three different methods to determine if a food allergy has been outgrown. The first is carefully asking and evaluating whether there have been any accidental exposures and how long the child has been completely reaction-free. The next method is monitoring food-specific IgE antibody levels from RAST blood tests. This may be the best predictor of whether it may be time to try to reintroduce the allergy-related food. If food-specific IgE antibody levels have decreased and your child has not had a reaction in over a year, your allergist may suggest a food or oral challenge, which is the last and final test. That involves feeding your child—under medical supervision in a hospital—the food that has caused reactions in the past to see if the allergy is still present or if no allergic reaction occurs. Such a challenge may include a placebo step to ensure the reaction is real. Placebo-controlled oral challenges may be single-blinded, meaning the person does not know exactly what is being taken, or double-blinded, meaning the person and the caregiver administering the challenge do not know what is being taken. However, many oral challenges do not include a placebo step and are considered "open," where all people involved know what is being taken. Many doctors think the food challenge is not only the best method of determining whether the allergy is gone but also the best way to safely reintroduce that food.

ADVICE TO HELP NONALLERGIC SIBLINGS

Some children have a hard time coping with the needs of their allergic siblings. They may feel resentment or jealously over "special treatment" given to their brother or sister, such as when safe treats are offered or when food-allergy accommodations dictate when and where to dine away from home.

To help offset these feelings, let your nonallergic children know how much their cooperation means to the well-being of the entire family. If an event comes up that you know will require special planning for food allergies, create opportunities then or at other

WILL A SIBLING DEVELOP FOOD ALLERGIES?

There is about a 7 percent likelihood that a sibling of a child who is allergic to peanuts will develop an allergy to peanuts. More generally, children with a sibling who has a food allergy are more likely to develop an atopic disease such as dermatitis, asthma, allergic rhinitis, and/or food allergies.

times for your nonallergic child to feel important, too. For instance, you can carve out one-on-one time away from the home with your nonallergic child where he or she can enjoy foods that are usually off-limits. But, more important, that's a good time to give him or her your undivided attention.

Encourage your children to help their sibling manage his or her food allergy. Here are some ways to enlist their help:

- Teach children why their brother or sister must avoid certain food. For example, even a very young child can be taught that milk gives big brother itchy bumps or makes his stomach hurt. If the sibling is older, teach him or her how to recognize symptoms of an allergic reaction and how to help if he or she thinks a reaction might be occurring.

- Assign tasks that promote teamwork among siblings, such as helping an adult prepare food or going grocery shopping. Older siblings can help by giving ingredient labels a first read-through, while at home younger children can place colorful "Safe" stickers on packaged foods that have been carefully checked to make sure they are allergen-free.

- Teach your nonallergic children ways to motivate their sibling to help with food-allergy management. For example, they could remind their brother or sister to ask if a food is safe before eating it or participate in role-play scenarios to help their sibling learn how to turn down food.

- I rewarded my own label-reading, conscientious child with a personal, dorm-size, mini-refrigerator in her room at age 8. I encouraged her to stock it with allergy-safe treats we purchase at the supermarket after she determined they were safe. This provided her with an incentive to manage her own allergy-safe diet from a young age. She even stores extra nibbles for siblings and friends who want to share the same goodies!

Finally, remind your children that each and every person is an individual, whether he or she has food allergies or not. All of our differences make us unique, and that should be valued. It can be difficult when one family member is ill, but part of family life is supporting each other regardless of the circumstances.

Not every suggestion listed here will apply to your family. It's best to use your own judgment about whether each child is old enough to take on a role in helping out with family food-allergy management or is willing to do so. While children may be enlisted to *help*, they should not feel as though managing a sibling's food allergy is solely their responsibility. It's a shared responsibility for all family members.

SHARING THE DIAGNOSIS
BEYOND YOUR IMMEDIATE FAMILY

Sharing your child's diagnosis of food allergy with other family members and your inner circle is never easy. It's not possible to assume that family and friends will remember to avoid reaction-causing foods right after you've told them about your child's allergy. They don't live with your child's allergy every single day, and they aren't in the habit of checking every label every time. You may need to remind them every once in a while until they become your most reliable and trusted food-allergy gatekeepers for birthday parties, playdates, even trips to the movie theater. Until then, remind yourself that it's natural to feel frustrated when those closest to you are still trying to get on board but may be forgetting or are not as empathetic as you'd like. This is a process that takes time, and, while your newly found vigilance may come easily to you, it's easy for others to initially forget and sometimes even misunderstand. There will be hurdles to overcome at school and at birthday parties, and worst of all there may be scorn and disbelief from some.

In the meantime, teach your child that when he or she is not sure about a food that a well-meaning grandmother or best friend offers, he or she needs to say, "No, thank you!" until you have a strategy in place and everyone is used to the food-allergy diagnosis. It might help to bring family members and live-in or routine caretakers to doctor appointments as you learn about your child's symptoms and continuing care. Be sure to ask your doctor if the allergy might change over time, and always keep medications up to date. Both over-the-counter antihistamines as well as epinephrine auto injectors have an expiration date, after which their effectiveness diminishes.

5

Schools and Camps

Let's be honest here: For parents, sending your child with life-threatening food allergies off at an early age to day care, preschool, or elementary school can be terrifying. Accidental ingestion of the offending allergen occurs most often at school, and a 2001 study published by *Archives of Pediatrics and Adolescent Medicine* states that one in five children with food allergies will have a reaction while in school. Younger elementary school students with an undiagnosed food allergy may experience their first food-allergy reaction at school.[1] Yikes!

Before you entrust your child to any school situation, you must educate your child about his or her food allergy at a level that is age appropriate. Make sure your child:

- Can distinguish between safe and unsafe foods.

- Has strategies for avoiding unsafe foods, such as never trading foods and not eating foods with unknown ingredients outside a designated dining area.

- Is aware of symptoms of his or her allergic reaction.

School is understandably a high-risk setting due to such factors as a large number of students, increased exposure to food allergens, as well as cross-contamination of tables, desks, and other surfaces. High-risk areas include the cafeteria and bus transportation for field trips, and high-risk activities include food sharing, hidden ingredients in prepared foods, fundraisers, bake sales, classroom parties and holiday celebrations, and craft, art, and science projects. There's also the issue of substitute teaching staff being unaware of the food-allergic student.

The school administration knows that allergic reactions to foods vary among students and can range from mild to severely life threatening. Ingestion of the food allergen is the principal route of exposure, though some very sensitive students may react to just touching or inhaling the allergen. The amount of food needed to trigger a reaction depends on multiple variables. Each food-allergic person's level of sensitivity may fluctuate over time. Not every ingestion exposure will result in anaphylaxis, though that potential always exists. For some, consumption of as little as one five-thousandth of a teaspoon of an allergy-causing food can, on rare occasions, prove fatal.

School is one area in food-allergy management that has shown tremendous improvement over the years. School districts and private schools recognize that because of the life-threatening nature of these allergies and their increasing prevalence, the administration needs to be on point and ready to care for students with food allergies. Today, school districts expect to have students with food allergies, and most schools are equipped and prepared to deal with food allergies and the potential for anaphylaxis. Many schools have action plans and make sure that staff are knowledgeable about preventive measures and are well prepared to handle even severe allergic reactions. They know this can save the life of your child.

In order to provide food-allergy education and establish related policies in schools, the Commonwealth of Massachusetts Department of Education established a task force in 2002 that presented to elementary school administrations the following hypothetical scenarios, prepared by Commissioner of Education Dr. David P. Driscoll, to help educate teachers and staff.

> *"A student with a milk allergy walks near the cafeteria where milk is being steamed and inhales the airborne milk protein, which causes hives, swelling, and respiratory distress."*

> *"A student with a peanut allergy is in his classroom and complains of itchy, swollen eyes and a tight chest only to discover later that the arts and crafts products in the classroom contain peanuts."*

This level of in-school education and awareness was literally unheard of before 2002 and needs to be mandated nationally. Schools are rising to the task of working closely with families and recognizing that for students at risk for food-induced allergy and anaphylaxis, the most important aspect of management in the school setting is *prevention*. Schools also better understand that raising a child with food allergies is challenging at home and that we as parents must ensure strict food avoidance, understand food labeling, and be on constant alert to implement an emergency medical plan at any given moment.

The fact is that parents of children with food allergies have crafted inventive ways to keep our children safe in a world that is not food-allergic friendly. Developing your child's own personal Food Allergy Action Plan is a concrete step to help ensure your child's safety when he or she is at school. This emergency care plan should detail your child's specific allergic reaction, specific symptoms, and the specific treatment you wish the school to seek. The Food Allergy Action Plan should clearly outline exactly what you want, and it's critical to have it signed by your child's physician. There's a particularly practical, useful, comprehensive Food Allergy Action Plan template you can easily download from the www.foodallergy.org website at no cost. It's easy to customize it yourself to suit your child's personal situation. A few schools have worked behind the scenes in order to develop their own action plan for allergic students. The schools in Massachusetts, for example, understand that the school + parent relationship is in the best interests of the student. School boards are cognizant that when a child begins elementary school, there must be trust and open dialogue between the school and the parents because what has worked so well at home is now being entrusted to unfamiliar people—strangers—some of whom are knowledgeable about food allergies and supportive of parents and others who are not. With an empathetic approach, these schools help parents and their children make the vital transition of moving from the safety of the home environment into the expanding world of the school—the real world. When the team sticks together, this provides one of the greatest lessons a child can learn: They are safe in the world outside their own home.

Schools can provide invaluable resources to children with food allergies and their families by helping the children feel accepted within the school community. They can teach children to:

- Keep themselves safe.

- Ask for help and learn to trust peers.

- Develop healthy and strong friendships.

- Acquire social skills.

- Accept more responsibility.

- Improve their self-esteem.

- Increase their self-confidence.

SAMPLE GUIDELINES AND LETTERS

The following resources were developed by the Massachusetts Department of Education for use in that state. They are excellent examples of how to protect food-allergic children in elementary schools.

Sample of School District Food-Allergy Protocols and Guidelines

Cafeteria Protocols/Guidelines

- What is the process for identifying students with life-threatening allergies?

- Is there a need for an allergen-free table?

- Which personnel will have responsibility for cleaning the tables, trays, and other facilities?

- What type of cleaning solution should be used?

- Who will provide training for cafeteria staff?

- Have the cafeteria monitors been informed?

Classroom Protocols/Guidelines

- Have all teachers, aides, volunteers, substitutes, and students been educated about food allergies?

- Have all parents/guardians of students in the class been notified that there is a student with a life-threatening food allergy and what foods must not be brought to school?

- Are there guidelines for allowable foods for lunch, snacks, parties, and so on?

- If not, who will establish these guidelines?

- Is there an allergen-free table/desk in the student's classroom?

- What are the cleaning protocols for this area?

- What type of cleaning solution should be used?

- Is there an understanding that classroom project materials containing the allergen may not be used?

- Have all students been taught proper hand-washing techniques before and after eating?

Environmental Protocols/Guidelines

• What is the school policy for the presence of animals?

• Is there an awareness of multiple and related allergies?

• What are the cleaning protocols for various areas of the school where allergens may be found?

Field Trip/School Bus Protocols/Guidelines

• How will the school nurse be notified about field trips in a timely manner?

• How will the child's Food Allergy Action Plan be communicated to responsible personnel on field trips, on the school bus, and in after-school programs? (All issues relating to the classroom and environment should be reviewed as appropriate for these situations.)

• Is the location of the field trip assessed to be safe for the student with allergies?

• Who will be trained to administer the epinephrine should an emergency occur? Is there a need for a registered nurse or aide to accompany the student?

• Should the student with allergies be seated near the driver, teacher, or advisor?

• Is there a no-food policy for the bus? Is it enforced?

• Do personnel have a system for communicating (such as cell phone or walkie-talkies)?

Custodial Protocols/Guidelines

• What cleaning solution is used?

• How often are the areas cleaned?

Emergency Response Protocols/Guidelines

- Have all school personnel received education about life-threatening allergic conditions?

- Has the school registered with the local Department of Public Health to train unlicensed personnel to administer epinephrine by auto injector?

- What specific personnel will be trained in the administration of epinephrine?

- Who will do the training?

- Will the parents be involved in the training?

- When will this training occur?

- What is the content of the training?

- How often will it be repeated during the school year? (Once, twice?)

- Where will the list of trained personnel be kept?

- Have local emergency medical services been informed, and has planning occurred to ensure the fastest possible response?

- Does the local emergency medical system carry epinephrine, and are they permitted to use it?

- When and how often are drills for such things as fire, earthquakes, hurricanes, and tornadoes part of the districtwide emergency response plan?

- In what unlocked area will epinephrine be stored?

- Where is the backup supply?

- Is it appropriate for this student to carry his/her own auto injector?

Sample of School District Food Allergy Letter
for Classmates and Parents

• If the parent agrees, since food allergies are a confidential health condition, a letter should be sent home with classmates to inform families of the school's peanut/nut or other food-allergy policy.

• A letter should be written on school stationery by a school nurse, teacher, and/or principal. Parents may help in composing the letter, but it must come from the school.

• The school nurse, teacher(s), and/or principal should sign the letter.

• Include a cut-off portion for parents of classmates to return to the school so that the staff is aware that the parents of classmates have received the information.

Date:

Dear Parents,

This letter is to inform you that a student in your child's classroom has a severe peanut/nut allergy. Strict avoidance of peanut/nut products is the only way to prevent a life-threatening allergic reaction. We are asking your assistance in providing the student with a safe learning environment.

If exposed to peanuts/nuts, the student may develop a life-threatening allergic reaction that requires emergency medical treatment. The greatest potential for exposure at school is to peanut products and nut products. To reduce the risk of exposure, the classroom will be peanut/nut free. Please do not send any peanut- or nut-containing products for your child to eat during snacktime in the classroom. Any exposure to peanuts or nuts through contact or ingestion can cause a severe reaction. If your child has eaten peanuts or nuts prior to coming to school, please be sure your child's hands have been thoroughly washed prior to entering the school.

Since lunch is eaten in the cafeteria, your child may bring peanut butter, peanut, or nut products for lunch. In the cafeteria there will be a designated peanut-free table where any classmate without peanut or nut products can sit. If your child sits at this table with a peanut or nut product, s/he will be asked to move to another table. This plan will help to maintain safety in the classroom while allowing non-allergic classmates to enjoy peanut/nut products in a controlled environment. Following lunch, the children will wash their hands prior to going to recess (or returning to the class). The tables will be cleaned with soap, water, and paper towels after each lunch.

We appreciate your support of these procedures. Please complete and return this form so that we are certain that every family has received this information. If you have any questions, please contact me.

x _____
    Signature of Principal / Teacher / Nurse

I have read and understand the peanut/nut-free classroom procedures. I agree to do my part in keeping the classroom peanut- and nut-free.

Child's Name: _____

Parent's Signature: _____

Date: _____

Sample of School District Food Allergy Letter for Substitute Teachers

Substitute teachers are an important link in the school staff. They must be included in the information chain regarding safety measures designed to protect the students with food allergies whom they supervise. Substitute teachers must receive written information that students with food allergies are in the class, information about peanut-free tables or other special modifications, and the resources available if a student has an allergic reaction. Here is a sample letter that teachers can leave with their lesson plans for a substitute:

Dear Substitute Teacher,

The students listed below in this class have severe life-threatening food allergies.

Please maintain the food-allergy avoidance strategies that we have developed to protect these students, which are attached. Should a student ingest, touch, or inhale the substance to which they are allergic (the allergen), a severe reaction (anaphylaxis) may follow requiring the administration of epinephrine (EpiPen®).

The Allergy Action Plan, which states who has been trained to administer epinephrine, is located _____ _____. Epinephrine is a life-preserving medication and should be given in the first minutes of a reaction.

STUDENT   ALLERGIES

_____   _____

_____   _____

_____   _____

_____   _____

Please treat this information confidentially to protect the privacy of the students. Your cooperation is essential to ensure their safety. Should you have any question please contact:

School Nurse: _____,

or Principal: _____

Signed, _____
                     (Classroom Teacher)

WHAT TO DO WHEN YOUR CHILD'S SCHOOL
DOES NOT HAVE AN ALLERGY MANAGEMENT PLAN

Some school districts and elementary schools have well-developed, detailed policies and comprehensive protocols that provide exemplary care for students with life-threatening allergies. They have made the leap in understanding that, as with all children with special needs, it's important that students with food allergies are able to have equal access to education, as well as each and every education-related benefit.

Regrettably, not all school districts or elementary schools have such policies and protocols. In such situations, successfully transitioning your food-allergic child into elementary school can feel like an utterly exhausting, daunting, solo endeavor without the support, understanding, and compassion of your school administration. What's needed is a systematic planning and multidisciplinary team approach before children with life-threatening food allergies enter school.

When I discovered in the summer of 2009 that the school my daughter was scheduled to attend did not have this sort of policy, I decided to become pro-active. I served on the Board of Directors of FAAN, the Food Allergy & Anaphylaxis Network, based in Fairfax, Virginia, for two years, taking an especially keen interest in the issue of school safety for allergic children. In 2012, FAAN merged with the Food Allergy Initiative and became FARE, *Food Allergy Research and Education,* to better reflect its mission, which is "to ensure the safety and inclusion of individuals with food allergies while relentlessly seeking a cure."

FAAN was established in 1991 by parent Anne Muñoz-Furlong at a time when information about food allergies was more difficult to find. Anne's daughter had been diagnosed with both severe milk allergy and severe egg allergy, and founding FAAN was Anne's way of providing education and support to the many parents of allergic children who needed help managing food allergy in their family life. FARE continues to offer practical, comprehensive resources for school safety guidelines.

Surprisingly, only thirteen states have published food-allergy management guidelines, which, in addition to Massachusetts, include Arizona, Tennessee, and Washington, among others. You can easily search online for this type of detailed information. Both FARE and the state guidelines offer plenty of resources to help you set up reasonable protocols for managing your child's food allergies at school if no policy is yet in place.

In preparation for a meeting with the principal, director, or headmaster of the school, you first need to ask your allergist to sign a written Food Allergy Action Plan, described above, to give to school staff and caregivers. This will outline the specific treatment course they should follow in the event of an allergic reaction. The plan needs to include the recommendation that the school should have on hand at least one epinephrine auto injector, but ideally two in the event a second dose is needed.

Once you're prepared with an action plan and auto injectors for the school, it's time to meet *in person* with the principal, director, or headmaster during hours set aside for parents of children with medical and/or special needs to meet with administrators, usually about two weeks before school opens. If the administrator is not familiar with food allergies, you need to explain your child's allergy in great detail, supply all written medical information about it from your child's allergist, including your child's Food Allergy Action Plan, and provide medications for emergency use at school. The last is a good way to promote the school's comprehension of the seriousness of food allergy and one with which they may not be familiar. I always share a story about an allergic reaction, making sure to include how it was triggered, all the specific symptoms, and the emergency medical treatment that was needed.

The same type of grab-n-go bag you keep within arms' reach can be duplicated, so it's available at all times at your child's school. Epinephrine auto injectors should have a shelf life of one year, so always be certain to check the expiration date before giving the medical bag to the school. It's best to ensure that the expiration date is at least twelve months away, so you won't need to replace the injectors during the school year. Depending on your child's particular circumstances and your doctor's recommendation, you may want to give the school additional medications such as antihistamine and an asthma inhaler and spacer. Keep in mind, however, the first rule of thumb with food allergies: Epinephrine auto injectors are the first line of defense for treating a potentially life-threatening allergic reaction, and, if there is any doubt, all efforts should be directed toward its immediate use.

A balanced school environment is still possible without a food-allergy policy already in place, but it requires forming a partnership between you and a team of key individuals who include the administration, teachers and coaches, the school nurse, dietitian, classmates, and, most important, other parents. Cumulatively, all these individuals play a key role in food-allergy management and your child's well-being at school. In working with your team, it's critical for parents to recognize up front that some members might need additional time to learn about food allergy and the many steps needed to avoid food allergens in the school setting. Actions that are second nature to you, such as reading ingredient labels and remembering the life cycle of foods, are not immediately intuitive actions for others. Fortunately, because food allergy has become such an emerging health issue, many elementary schools have already adopted and implemented food-allergy management strategies, including safe zones. In some cases they even provide a completely allergen-free environment.

FARE and I recommend using the following very basic, broad, friendly checklist for schools without food-allergy policies and procedures. Even though the principal or head administrator may have briefed the entire staff about your child's allergy and handed out copies of your child's Food Allergy Action Plan, it's good to arrange ahead of time with the administrator that you would like to meet with selected members of your team, such as the teacher(s), nurse, and dietitian, who will have the most contact with your child throughout the school day, before the first day of school to:

- Introduce yourself and share information about your child.

- Find out what they already know about food allergy.

- Provide information on the basics (if necessary), clear up any misconceptions, and discuss the role team members play in managing your child's food allergy.

- Be sure everyone who is most likely to come in contact with your child during the school day has a copy of your child's Food Allergy Action Plan, and ask them to keep it in an easily accessible location.

- Discuss with members of your school team any additional types of written management plans they need to keep on file. Most often these include an individualized healthcare plan (IHP), which is recommended by the National Association of School Nurses (NASN) for students whose healthcare needs may affect their ability to attend school safely and perform academically. Also included may be a 504 Plan, which applies to students who have a disability that affects their ability to participate fully, alongside their peers, in all regular facets of the school day. Children whose food allergy may result in severe, life-threatening reactions, in the opinion of the child's allergist, meet the definition of disability under Section 504.7 of the Americans with Disabilities Act. Most school districts or systems should have a 504 coordinator who is available to help you develop a 504 Plan if you request one.

FARE Food Allergy School Checklist

Promoting food safety in the classroom is vitally important. Be sure to speak with your child's teacher about that. Then work with the teacher to establish and help implement the following strategies to avoid exposure to food allergens that might risk your child having an allergic reaction.

- Having a "no food sharing" or "no food trading" rule.

- Encouraging hand washing after all food handling and eating. Liquid soap, bar soap, and sanitizing wipes effectively clean hands of potential allergens, but antibacterial sanitizing gels do not.

- Washing all surfaces after food is prepared, eaten, or used. Commercial wipes and spray cleaners are most effective at removing allergen protein from tables and other surfaces.

- Using nonfood items for classroom projects, academic rewards, and classroom celebrations.

- Encouraging strict use of only packaged food items with ingredient labels, as opposed to home-baked goods.

- Avoiding modeling clay, paper mâché, crayons, soaps, and other materials that may contain allergens.

- Keeping safe snacks for your child in the classroom for unplanned events, along with safe, nonperishable meals in case lunch is compromised or in the event of a shelter-in-place emergency or evacuation to another location.

- Providing safe snacks for the entire class so everyone can eat what your child eats.

- Having students store their lunches in a specific location.

- Allowing you to become a "classroom parent," so you can have advance notice of planned activities that might involve food. Some classroom parents are chosen over the summer by the local Parent-Teacher Association. If you cannot be a classroom parent, ask to be invited to class events such as field trips, so you can help the teacher monitor your child's exposure to food allergens.

- Making sure a copy of your child's Food Allergy Action Plan is available for substitute teachers, along with the food-allergy letter to substitutes.

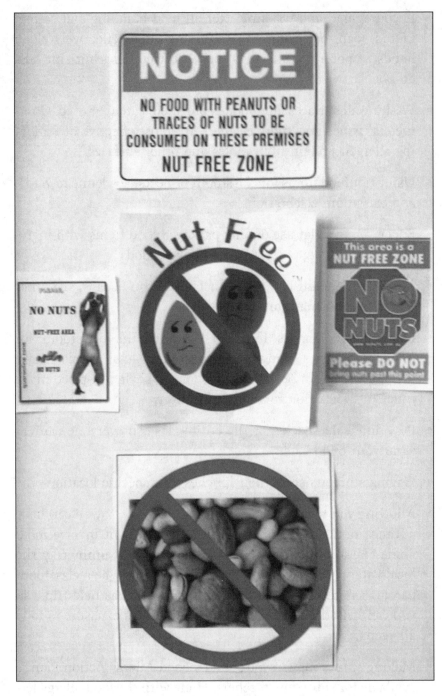

School safe zone signs in San Francisco, California.

- Sending a letter from the school informing classroom parents that there is a child in the class with a food allergy in order to raise awareness of food allergy and help reduce allergens in the classroom. Such a letter can help promote parental support of the food-allergy management team.

- Asking the school administration to designate your child's classroom as one that is not used for outside activities and events that involve food during nonschool hours. Taking this precaution will help reduce contamination of desks and other surfaces with food allergens when school is not in session.

KEEPING CLEAN AT SCHOOL

Since people with peanut allergy can have an allergic reaction to very small quantities of peanut allergen, scientists investigated how well different cleaning agents worked to remove particles of the peanut allergen. The test showed that simple measures of cleanliness can remove many allergens from the classroom environment. For example, simply washing your hands with liquid soap, bar soap, or commercial wipes was enough to remove peanut allergens, and common household cleaning agents, such as Formula 409®, Lysol® Sanitizing Wipes, and Target® cleaner with bleach, removed peanut allergen from such surfaces as tabletops, desks, and doorknobs.[2]

WHAT ABOUT SUMMER CAMPS AND FOOD ALLERGIES?

Summer camps present specific challenges for keeping children with food allergies safe. When considering sending your child to camp, it is essential to prepare ahead of time. It helps to consider the following issues:

- Should the camp be accredited by the American Camp Association? The benefit is that these camps are professionally reviewed and must meet certain standards. (Only 30 percent of U.S. camps are currently accredited.) To learn more about accreditation standards and to help locate an appropriate camp for your child, you may want to check out www.acacamps.org.

- Does the camp have a policy for managing food-allergic children?

- Does the camp have a health team (physicians, nurses, or other personnel) designated to take responsibility in an emergency? What are the person's credentials?

- How far is the camp from an emergency facility? If it's in a rural area, does that facility have a doctor on call and/or is there emergency medical transportation or 911 service?

- Will medications to treat an allergic reaction be kept in a safe, easily accessible place?

- Will your camper be outside the camp (at a lake, on an overnight campout, on a bike, or on hiking trails)? If so, what emergency plan will be in place?

- How will the camp communicate a child's food-allergy information to essential personnel—the child's counselor, activity leaders, kitchen coordinator?

- How will the camp help prevent accidental ingestions? Will precautions be provided such as food labeling in the dining area, creating safe meals for a trip or cookout, storing safe snacks in cabins, and avoiding allergens in craft areas?

- What plan will be in place in the dining hall by food service personnel to ensure that your child will eat safely? How will they be educated about creating a safe meal?

Once you have located the best summer camp for your child, it's time to meet with the camp director and the camp's primary healthcare person to discuss your child's allergy. Here are some questions to ask:

- Does the camp have previous experience with food-allergic campers?

- Does the camp application and/or health form allow you to fully describe your child's food allergy, including his or her Food Allergy Action Plan?

- What is the response time for local emergency medical teams when 911 is called?

- Is anyone trained to use an auto injector? If not, will the health-care person be trained?

- What is the camp's medication policy? Does it include labels on all medications and extra doses? Does your child need to carry his or her own grab-n-go bag?

- How will the staff be notified about your child's allergy and instructed in how to deal appropriately with it and any potential allergic reactions?

- Will the camp contact you if your child has a reaction?

Suggested Guidelines for Family, Camper, and Camp

Once you are satisfied that the camp is able to properly care for your food-allergic child, you'll need to prepare your family and your camper for it. The Boy Scouts of America have excellent policies and guidelines for its "Patriots' Path Council" summer camp operations in New Jersey. The Boy Scout Council adopted the American Association of Camp Nurses (AACN) recommendations for allergies in camp, developed and written by FARE and reproduced here with permission. They clearly outline the family responsibility, the camper responsibility, and the camp's responsibility.

The Family Responsibility

Before camp:

- Become familiar with the camp's food-allergy plan.

- Meet with the food service staff.

- Identify a responsible adult or leader who is knowledgeable of camper's needs.

At check-in:

- Notify the camp of your Scout's allergies.

- Complete the form (attached) and present to the health officer with the medication (for review).

- Meet with the health officer.

- Discuss what happens if an exposure occurs and [the amount of] time to onset of symptoms.

- Ensure the form is complete, with contact information.

- Ensure medication has not expired/gone bad.

- Review proper use of EpiPen®.

The Camper Responsibility

Before camp:

- Become familiar with the camp's food-allergy plan.

- Become familiar with what food the camp serves and what alternatives are available.

At camp:

- NEVER trade food with other campers.

- Do NOT eat anything with unknown ingredients.

- Read ALL labels and check with an adult if it is appropriate to eat.

- Alert an adult/staff/health officer of ANY reaction, no matter how mild.

- Do NOT go off alone, especially if symptoms are beginning.

- Know alternate locations where it is safe to eat.

- Have awareness of potential allergen sources (kitchen, dining hall, trading post, etc.).

The Camp Responsibility

Before camp:

- Make available storage areas for food brought in by Scout/parents.

- Ensure all staff know how to contact the health officer/EMT.

- Be aware of emergency procedures for medical emergencies, including allergies.

- Be aware of the signs/symptoms of an allergic reaction, both mild and severe.

- Assure that the health officer has the proper training, including EpiPen® administration.

At camp:

- Ensure that Scouts with food allergies are safely included in camp activities (cooking and food-related activities).

- Be certain that all staff (especially food service staff) are aware of the campers with food allergies.

- Notify the health officer of any Scouts with signs/symptoms of food allergies, both mild and severe.

- Post "Allergen Zone" signage at key locations, including dining hall and trading post.

- Ensure medical history confidentiality of ALL Scouts and leader.

Camp is an important milestone in a young person's life. So ask the right questions, remind the camp staff regularly about your child's food allergy, take a deep breath, and let your child have fun!

PREPARING FOR COLLEGE

What about life after high school? As you and your college-bound teen begin to visit college campuses, you can check to see if prospective schools have disability offices. It's becoming increasingly common for colleges and universities to recognize that food-allergic students need special eating and medical accommodations. The top four issues to consider when making plans for your college student are housing, cafeteria and dining plans, transportation in the area for access to supermarkets and doctor appointments, and the college's emergency response plans. Some schools have their own private ambulance service and a campus security team, so make sure to check with them about how they would handle an allergic emergency. These years are vitally important so that your student is able to gain independence in the real world. While these challenges are scary at times, college life is a healthy component of young adulthood.

6

Restaurants

Where I reside in the Bay Area, aside from our stunning Fog City backdrop against the Golden Gate Bridge, San Francisco is best known as a foodie haven with great local cuisine. When moving to the Bay Area more than a decade ago, I didn't take into account the overwhelming presence of seafood in the city. It took some adjustments to be able to enjoy the beauty and culture and still dodge seafood, which seemed to be everywhere all at once. Between fragrant, buttery sautés of local salmon redolent from sidewalk cafes and the robust cioppinos and chowders all along Fisherman's Wharf and Pier 39, it has proven challenging to stay out of my danger zone. The most difficult facet about seafood allergy is that you can have severe allergic reactions even if you don't accidentally consume fish—simply by exposure to aerosolized fish protein in cooking vapors or steam. This means, in essence, you become allergic to air. So I have learned to carefully stay far away from steam tables or kitchen stove tops when seafood is being cooked. I avoid sushi and waterfront seafood restaurants entirely, even when well-meaning friends helpfully inform me, "The restaurant does serve a few other dishes!" It's too high risk because of the common use of fish and fish ingredients and almost certain cross-contamination even if you didn't order a seafood dish. This holds true for all Big 8 allergens in restaurants, and people living with food allergies must be particularly alert to what's on their plate.

Keeping control of your food's life cycle at a restaurant can be intimidating, especially when the kitchen is behind closed doors and you can't tell whether your waitperson understands exactly what you mean by "allergic to wheat." Nonetheless, learning how to eat out with food allergies is absolutely vital for your social experience, and it allows you much-needed downtime from your own kitchen. Over the years I've developed a tried-and-true safe list of restaurants, which are adept at expertly accommodating my needs, and I've even found several completely fish-free restaurants in and around San Francisco.

STEPS NEEDED TO DINE OUT SAFELY

The first step to dining out safely is performing some preliminary research on your own. Start by calling destinations you'd like to try in your area. You can brainstorm and get inspired by using two excellent national online resources for safe eating: www.Aller gyEats.com and www.AllerDine.com.

Then investigate restaurant websites and look for either a menu listing major ingredients or an email address where you can ask for information about specific recipes. Some restaurants opt to post their full, official allergy policy on their websites. For example, some major chains like Olive Garden even provide recipes online so you can find out exactly what ingredients are in the dishes on their menu.

If you want to find out what a restaurant's policy is on serving diners with food allergies, then you'll need to call the place well ahead of your dinner date. Be sure to provide as much notice as possible so the staff will have enough time to assess if they can keep you safe. Because the restaurant industry is particularly intense, it is good to place your phone call at the beginning of the workday, long before the hectic lunch rush and end-of-evening fatigue. If possible, call before or after the busy hours, say, between

2 and 4 p.m. Avoiding peak times when dining at the new restaurant is also recommended. Besides, you're far more likely to get attentive service, especially on your first few visits if you avoid the lunch and dinner rushes. Remember, time works in the food-allergic diner's favor at a restaurant, so nothing is rushed when checking on ingredients and following up with additional questions.

Questions to Ask a Restaurant

The following list of questions to ask a restaurant isn't all-inclusive. If you or your child have special concerns related to your particular allergies, make up your own list of questions to get the answers you need to eat safely.

- Do you have a formal allergy policy? Is the waitstaff educated and trained in handling food allergies?

- Do you have a book or list of ingredients in all foods you serve?

- Will you custom-prepare a meal for a food-allergic individual?

- What is your kitchen layout?

- What kind of oil is used in the fryer? If that oil is safe, what else is fried in it?

- Are there dedicated cooking surfaces that are kept safe for food-allergic cooking?

- Are cooking utensils for different foods kept separate and safe?

- Does the waitstaff know to keep food-allergy dishes away from other dishes? Do they know that allergens can't just be picked off a meal?

If you are not satisfied with any answer you are given when you call with questions, feel free to ask to speak to the manager or the chef, as they have more intimate knowledge of the many aspects of food service. If you are still not satisfied, you will need to continue to search for a safe restaurant in which to dine. A good rule of thumb: It's better to be told "no" by a restaurant after they have assessed their ability to cope with food allergies than to get a rushed, halfway "yes" and then succumb to your food allergy in the dining room. I've learned this rule the hard way. While I've never seen the inside of an ambulance, over the course of my life I've had to make dozens of seafood-related trips to the hospital to be evaluated and in some cases given an injection of prescription antihistamine.

Be intrepid yet responsible when dining somewhere new, and remember that communication is key. Learning how to dine out safely is mostly a matter of training oneself to ask lots and lots of questions. When you arrive at the restaurant, make sure to meet the manager and explain your condition thoroughly, reminding the establishment of your food allergy. Tell the manager that you would like to brief your designated waiter about your food allergy once you are seated—he or she is your vital liaison with the kitchen.

When you are looking over the menu, remember to be mindful of hidden allergens lurking in breading, salad dressing, complex sauces, garnishes, or certain courses. Most restaurants are pre-pared and equipped for food-allergic diners, and you've certainly done your best to alert them to your medical condition, yet you can't let your guard down completely. Sometimes products used by chefs, such as mixes for sauces or dressings, list ingredients by alternate names. So if you request that something be left out of or off a dish, it's vital to know all the terms, including derivatives, under which your allergen may be listed (see Chapter 2, The Big 8 Allergy-Causing Foods).

Allergy-friendly options on restaurant menus fall into two cat-egories: dishes that do not include your allergen and dishes that include your allergen as a condiment or garnish that can easily not be placed on your plate. In many restaurants, the second cat-egory predominates, so consider suggesting substitutions to your waiter. For example, someone who is allergic to milk might ask,

"With my food allergy, is it possible for the chef to prepare the risotto without milk or cheese?"

I always check with the waitstaff and chef to ensure fish is not cooked in the same skillet or in the same oil as other food items. It's also good to make sure your dishes are not prepared with the same utensils or on the same work surfaces as your allergen, or you will be subject to cross-contamination. One savvy chef taught me years ago to tell a waiter, "I am also severely allergic to *utensils* that have touched fish." That has more impact, yes? However, two avenues of cross-contamination are difficult to avoid. The first is restaurant grills. So always inquire whether a food marinated in an allergen is cooked directly on the same grill as any grilled dish you may want to order. The second is frying oil. If you are allergic to something cooked in a deep fryer, you have to avoid eating anything else fried in that oil.

When your meal arrives, trust your instincts. If you have doubts about your order after you've received it, it's perfectly fine to politely ask your waiter to double-check with the kitchen. Then do not feel shy or embarrassed about sending food back if it turns out a mistake has been made. Simply removing the allergenic items from your plate isn't sufficient to keep you safe. If the meal does contain an allergen, you must be brought an entirely new meal.

FROM THE RESTAURANT'S PERSPECTIVE: HOW TO SAFELY SERVE GUESTS WITH FOOD ALLERGIES

While most people reading this book are probably not planning on opening a food-allergy-sensitive restaurant, you might find it useful to give the following list of how to safely serve customers with food allergies to a receptive restaurant that doesn't already have a safe food-allergy policy or procedures. Reviewing the list might also help you come up with questions that directly address your or your child's safety needs. Since levels of sensitivity vary, it is absolutely important that restaurants prevent contact between known allergens and the food-allergic guest's meal. Remember, if a single protein from the food allergen comes into contact with the guest's meal that could trigger an allergic reaction.

- **Communication is key.** If a guest mentions that he or she has a food allergy, take the person seriously. Have the server inform either the manager or the person on staff with food-allergy knowledge.

- **Have someone on staff who knows about food allergies.** Though it is important that all staff know the basics of food allergies, make sure each shift has someone who has extensive knowledge of both the menu and different allergens, so he or she can help guests select menu items that will not cause an allergic reaction.

- **Avoid cross-contamination.** Cross-contamination occurs when food proteins mix through either direct or indirect contact. Food allergens can be transferred via unclean hands or utensils, preparation surfaces, fryer vats, and even garnishes. Remember, it may only take a single protein to cause an allergic reaction.

- **Cleaning and sanitization.** Any surfaces used for preparation and service of meals need to be properly cleaned and sanitized. For preparation areas, the work surface and all utensils, pots, and pans need to be washed with hot soapy water—soap must be used because it deactivates the protein causing the allergy. All work-surface areas, counters, and cutting surfaces need to be cleaned thoroughly between uses. Adopting a color-coded cutting board system helps minimize the risk of cross-contamination when preparing foods. Here are two examples of ways to avoid cross-contamination:

  - After using a food slicer to slice cheese, the slicer must be cleaned thoroughly before being used to slice other foods to prevent contamination with cheese protein.

  - Wash trays or cookie sheets after each use as oils can seep through wax paper or other liners and contaminate the next food cooked on the sheet or tray.

- **Prepare food separately.** To prevent cross-contamination, use separate utensils, different preparation areas, and maybe even separate equipment if necessary to keep allergens from contacting specially prepared foods.

- **Serve the dish separately.** Cross-contact can occur when prepared meals are being carried to the table, so be sure to carry a specially prepared meal separately from other dishes.

- **Check with the guest immediately to ensure everything is satisfactory.** With food-allergic customers, it is important to ensure that no allergic reaction occurs once they begin eating. So have the waitperson swing by their table a few minutes after serving to ask if everything is all right. This will further show that the restaurant cares about the customer's health, and that contact might help the waitperson spot a reaction early on, rather than the customer having to flag down the server.

- **Do not include hidden ingredients.** Though you do not have to give out your entire preparation process, mentioning the eight most common allergen ingredients on the menu will be helpful to guests with allergies.

- **Mention any menu changes.** When changing ingredients in a dish, be sure to immediately make the change on the menu and let guests know that the dish contains different ingredients to which they may be allergic.

- **Have alternate dishes and ingredients on hand.** Several substitutions can be used to replace common food allergens without changing the flavor of the meal.

- **If you do not know about ingredients, say so.** If a guest with food allergies is considering a certain dish, and you are not certain if the ingredients contain an allergen, say so. In all instances regarding customer health, it is better to be safe than sorry.

- **Call 911 immediately if an allergic reaction occurs.** If a customer says he or she is having an allergic reaction, do not wait to see if the symptoms pass. Allergic reactions can be life threatening, so call 911 immediately and have servers notify management immediately.

THE BIG 8 AT THE RESTAURANT BAR

For adults managing food allergies at a restaurant, food is far from the only concern. Food allergens such as milk, soy, and tree nuts may also be found in many cocktails at the restaurant bar or served at your table. Wheat is prevalent in many beers. Aside from being vigilant about ingredients in beverages, adults managing food allergies must also use caution when drinking alcoholic beverages to ensure that their judgment is not negatively affected and that their ability to make decisions, recognize an allergic reaction quickly, and administer medication is not impaired. Alcohol can also influence how quickly a food allergen is absorbed by the body, resulting in symptoms occurring at a faster pace.

Here's a list of some allergy-causing ingredients that may be hidden in alcoholic drinks.

- Tree nuts in some specialty beers (particularly seasonal ales)
- Hazelnuts in Frangelico
- Milk in Irish Cream
- Egg used to create froth on the top of some cocktails
- Almonds in Amaretto and also in several brands of gin
- Milk in white chocolate liqueurs

If you're planning on drinking alcohol at the restaurant bar or at your table, it's good to remain mindful of the cross-contamination potential with cocktail shakers and stirrers. Also keep a keen eye out when garnishes are used on cocktails.

TREAT AN ACCOMMODATING RESTAURANT
LIKE A BEST FRIEND

Many restaurants and their staff will touch you deeply with their willingness to help you enjoy the dining experience. Some have gone so far to accommodate the allergic patron that they have created an "allergy key" in the restaurant's electronic billing system that prints out information in bold red letters at the top of the diner's ticket. As part of the restaurant's food-allergy protocol, the food-allergic diner's plate may be lined with an additional plate beneath it, as a physical reminder that this meal is being prepared for a food-allergic guest.

Treat this unique and special category of restaurant like you would a true blue friend. Bring the restaurant as much business as you can, tell friends about it, and thank the place sincerely for the exemplary service it provides. Hand deliver a note or card the day after a memorable meal; it's sure to brighten up the staff's work environment. It's a great pleasure to be able to walk into a dining establishment where you know that your medical needs will remain low key and yet be completely attended to. For example, here's a special shout-out to former sous chef Brent at Spruce Restaurant who has gone above and beyond for many years to happily provide me with a social experience and atmosphere in which I can enjoy fine dining safely!

7

Transportation and Family Vacations

Traveling can be hazardous to your health, especially if you're food allergic. Enclosed spaces on planes, trains, and automobiles leave little escape from the Big 8. Regardless of the distance you're traveling, it is important to think about your or your loved one's restricted diet, especially the first few times you travel after a food-allergy diagnosis. It won't take long, however, to become a pro.

Food Allergy Travel Packing List

Begin with a food-allergy travel packing list. What you need to carry with you depends on how long you'll be en route and whether you'll have access to a kitchen and a grocery store at your destination.

- Your medical grab-n-go bag and any other doctor-prescribed medication.

- A cooler filled with prepared safe foods, snacks, and utensils if traveling by train or automobile.

- A carry-on bag filled with prepared safe foods, snacks, and utensils if traveling by airplane.

- Additional safe foods, ideally dry foods, that can be boxed, packed away, or even mailed ahead.

- Contact information for a local allergist and directions to the hospital closest to your destination. The website UCompare HealthCare.com can help you find a qualified doctor if you don't have a recommendation in the area.

TRAVELING BY AIRPLANE AND TRAIN

Airlines are accustomed to dealing with all Big 8 food allergies. The most problematic allergy when flying is severe peanut allergy because of the possibility of a reaction from inhaled peanut dust within the enclosed area that has only recirculated airflow. Some airlines have stopped serving peanut snacks during flights to avoid this possibility, and some will even request over the public address system that passengers refrain from eating peanuts. Virtually all airlines stress that they cannot guarantee a truly peanut-free flight because it's impossible to control what snacks passengers carry with them.

Here are a series of steps that will help keep you or your child safe during airplane travel.

1. Before you travel, talk to your allergist about your particular risks of an inhalation reaction. In most cases, this risk is low, and your primary concern will be avoiding allergens in food you eat on board the airplane. Nonetheless, your doctor is the best person to advise you on this issue. If you think it would be helpful, ask your doctor to sign a letter (which you can write based on the school food allergy plan) detailing your or your child's food allergy and how best to handle it while traveling.

2. If possible, select your flight time wisely and strategically. Some airlines recommend early morning travel because airplane interiors have a designated cleaning after the last flight of the previous day. Ask about particularly full flights, as a less crowded

option will offer you a natural buffer zone away from other passengers.

3. Notify the airline of your food allergies at the time when you make your reservation. You will also need to follow up again on the day of your flight. If you are booking an online reservation, some forms have a place to indicate any medical and/or special needs. If your online form doesn't have that section, you will need to email or call the airline's customer service hotline to explain your food allergy and provide the hotline representative with your flight and seat numbers. Ask if the airline is amenable to avoiding serving snacks that trigger your medical condition; some are willing.

4. Make certain you read the airline's written policy about allergies before traveling. If you have any additional questions or seek clarity, call the customer relations hotline well before travel to ensure everything will be safe for you.

5. Though flight attendants should already have your family's food-allergy information on a dietary-needs list, it might be helpful to identify yourself upon boarding to confirm that attendants are aware of your medical condition and needs. Once on board, be certain to have your grab-n-go bag in your carry-on luggage. Keep your medical bag in your lap or directly beneath your seat at your feet. Speak with flight attendants to see if they will make any announcements to ensure your flight is allergy-safe. In addition, be alert to passengers who are eating snacks in close proximity to you.

6. In the event of a reaction, immediately inform the flight attendants as you simultaneously begin administering treatment. If you need help, the flight crew will solicit assistance from any qualified medical personnel who may be on board, and the crew is trained to assist you with cardiopulmonary resuscitation (CPR) or oxygen, if necessary. As always with any allergic reaction, remain as calm as possible. Although you will be in the

air, it's good to reassure yourself that you have rescue medication in hand and qualified personnel will assist you.

Closely follow the same guidelines for airline travel when traveling by train. Notify the train company of your food allergies at the time you make your reservation. Amtrak has best practices to keep all travelers safe, but it does serve foods with peanuts and peanut oils. The company recommends you bring your own food for train travel and allows travelers to bring a cooler on board. Meals are served in dining cars, but the lounge car has a snack bar, complete with chips, drinks, and packaged nuts. Passenger cars and cars with roomettes are usually removed from dining and lounge cars, but, if you have a severe peanut allergy, it's always a good practice to sit in a car that is distant from these cars. Another good rule to follow is, if you can smell the strong scent of your allergen, it means that airborne particles are entering your nose and lungs, so it's always best to keep a safe distance from overwhelming odors.

While some people have no choice but to travel economically, those with strong food allergies who are subject to airborne contamination need to consider if they can risk the chance of riding a crowded bus where people bring their own food.

TRAVELING BY CAR

If you're traveling via your own transportation, it's easy enough to store food and snacks in the car. Your cooler, packed with ice and all your favorite foods, is an essential travel item, which helps by providing both variety and convenience. But there's every chance you'll make pit stops at mini-markets and restaurants. While it will take advance planning for a lengthy road trip, it pays to do research to find allergy-aware chain restaurants along the highway. Checking online and following up with phone calls as recommended in Chapter 6, Restaurants, will help you locate allergy-safe restaurants along the way. Happy trails to you!

TAKING FAMILY VACATIONS

Whether it's a Park Hopper pass at Disneyland or the getaway of a lifetime to Paris, vacations present a great opportunity to create memories and enjoy rich new experiences. With your food allergy, you may worry that what should be a relaxing break could become a dangerous adventure. Just as you notified your transportation carrier in advance about your food allergy, it's good to similarly plan ahead with your hotel, resort, or host. Taking precautions is key.

First, notify your hotel or host of your food allergies at the time when you make your reservation or accept an invitation. At that time, inquire about any policies for food-allergic guests, and ask if your hotel accommodations include in-room kitchens or kitchenettes for your convenience. If so, you can pack your own pots, pans, and utensils; I do it every trip. You can bring your own food or send it ahead by mail, or take a quick trip to the local supermarket once you arrive, and voila!—allergy-safe dining in your own hotel room. At our favorite destination hotel, I even take our family's food-allergy safe meals on trays to the pool cabanas, and we blend right in. Because dealing with food allergies day to day takes a tremendous emotional and psychological toll on each of us, being able to sit among other families eating casually on a rooftop or poolside in the sunshine and fresh air helps the mind be "on vacation" as well.

Some hotels offer complimentary toiletries in miniature-sized bottles without ingredients listed on them. So when you're packing for your hotel or hosted stay, be certain to bring your own travel allergen-free soaps, shampoos, lotions, and toothpaste. Behind the scenes and ahead of time, you can request that the hotel mini-bar's packaged cookie, candy, and food snacks be removed prior to your arrival. Once at your destination, continue to personally carry your grab-n-go medical bag instead of handing it off to a bellhop. Identifying an easy-to-locate, designated place for your bag in your new quarters is a good idea; a safe place might be on the bedside table. With careful planning, there will no doubt be blissful times when your food-allergy worries will melt away in your allergy-safe vacation hideaway. Enjoy those moments.

If you're traveling to a destination for a wedding or other significant occasion where food is being prepared and served by a catering company, asking your hosts to arrange allergy-safe dishes is not recommended. They are no doubt making multiple behind-the-scenes accommodations for a wide range of guests' preferences and needs. Although your hosts mean well, they are multitasking in the midst of a major life event, so asking for their help is the least efficient way to ensure you have safe food. Instead, early in the event-planning process, ask directly for the catering company's telephone number and speak to the company liaison or chef in advance so you can assess whether you will be able to eat safely at the event or if you should eat beforehand or pack a small, discreet energy snack in your bag. If necessary when you arrive at the event, make sure to find the head of the catering staff and explain your condition thoroughly in person, reminding them of your food allergy.

For any short-notice gathering, such as a memorial, it's best to simply assume that people are distracted, gathering hurriedly to pay respects, and the food is unsafe. If you must eat at an event of this nature, single-ingredient foods like fruit, vegetables, or cheese are the safest bets, assuming they do not trigger your allergies. For more about other special family events, see Chapter 8, Happy Holidays.

Special Precautions for Foreign Travel

If you are traveling to a foreign country and staying at a hotel where there is a language barrier, it helps to carry a card that explains what foods you can't eat in the local language. The website www.selectwisely.com has a wide selection of Food & Travel translation cards (please see page 88), which are excellent for communicating your food allergies and even for addressing the possi-

HIDDEN BIG 8 ALLERGENS
IN FOREIGN COUNTRIES

- **Milk** is used in many cakes (*leche*) and desserts in Spain.

- **Eggs** are found in fried rice dishes in China and chicken dishes in Ethiopia, while hard-boiled eggs are found in a favorite dish (*zebhi dorho*) in Eritrea.

- **Peanuts** are used in many dim sum dishes (*congee*) and hot mustard greens in China.

- **Tree nuts** such as ground almonds are used to replace flour in Spain, while almond paste and almond powder are present in pastries in Argentina and Portugal.

- **Wheat** is a common base for some beers in Germany (*Weisse*).

- **Soy** is used in cooking broths and sauces in China, and *miso,* made with soy paste, is widely found in Japanese soups and dishes.

- **Fish** is used in cooking broths and stirred into breakfast porridge in China and Japan.

- **Shellfish** is used in cooking broths and sauces in China and Japan.

bility of cross-contamination. Show this card to your server and, if possible, the chef at each and every restaurant you visit. A great place to store your card is in your grab-n-go bag, which you should have with you at all times on your trip.

In advance of your international trip, it's good to research regional cuisines in order to have a clear understanding of the dishes you'll want to avoid completely.

Take some time to learn the word for your allergen in the language of the country you're visiting. Practice it often and always make sure you can recognize the word in writing on food packaging.

Front

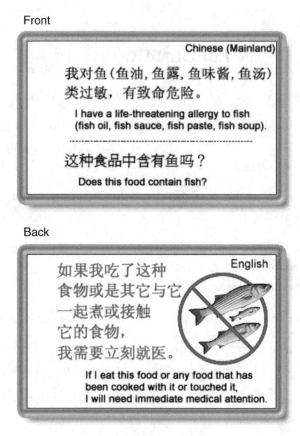

The website www.selectwisely.com has an impressive range of affordable and easy-to-order international language cards for food-allergic travelers.

Do your best, but also be aware that food-labeling laws in many other countries differ greatly from those in the United States. So don't be afraid to ask questions, show your Food & Travel translation card, and when in doubt: Just say no. With diligent planning, the best part of your foreign travel will be engaging with the local people, the culture, and—when it's possible to share safely—the cuisine.

8

Happy Holidays

Holidays are a particularly challenging time for us food-allergic individuals with so many desserts and homemade treats, casseroles, and dips all without ingredient labels. They may also prove difficult for food-allergic children who can feel left out of the traditional festivities, many of which center around food. Hosts may also feel challenged by food allergies, as they frequently must tend to a wide range of preferences and needs behind the scenes. All the excitement makes it more difficult to be informed about the life cycle of each and every food. Usually a call to a manufacturer of holiday candies will alleviate your concern, but, if you are unable to verify all ingredients and allergens, then dispose of the snacks and the candy.

SIX SEASONAL HOLIDAYS

Most people think of kids when they think of seasonal holidays like Halloween, but in reality everybody enjoys Valentine's Day, Thanksgiving, and the spring and year-end religious holidays. Here are some tips for getting through the holidays while staying happy, healthy, and allergy-free.

Valentine's Day

February has been the month to celebrate love for a long time, dating back to the Middle Ages. Legend has it that St. Valentine was an imprisoned man who fell in love with his jailor's daughter, and he sent the first card himself when he wrote her a letter and signed it "Your Valentine," words still traditionally used on cards today. Perhaps we'll never know the true identity and story behind the man named St. Valentine, but this much is certain: Students anticipate the annual tradition of exchanging Valentine cards, and often these notes come with candy. Like other seasonal candies, Valentine sweets are often not produced in regular manufacturing facilities, so read all labels carefully. Many miniature candies don't have an ingredient label. Of course, unwrapped candies loose in a card are a complete no-no. It's critical for parents of younger children with food allergies to caution them against eating candy unless it has been preapproved. Dairy-free and nut-free chocolates often look and taste like most other candies, so children, from a very young age onward, need to be aware that their candy is different and allergy-safe.

A Safe and Successful Valentine's Day Classroom Checklist

In classrooms everywhere, elementary school teachers and room parents plan festive, cheerful Valentine's Day parties for their students each year. This is a time when schools and parents need to work closely together to keep their guard up due to the potential for food-allergy reactions as the excitement level runs high and snacks abound. The following FARE Food Allergy Valentine Checklist provides some helpful reminders for the school as this holiday approaches.

- Call the teacher or the room parent (whoever is taking the lead on organizing the party) to remind him or her about your child's food allergies and discuss how your child can participate in the event safely alongside his or her classmates.

- Reinforce safety rules with your child about not accepting foods that have not been cleared by you or another designated adult.

- Remind your child not to open any Valentine's Day candies from classmates.

- If it's not too late, perhaps suggest some games and easy crafts that can be done during the party in lieu of eating food in the classroom.

- Work out a plan with your child's teacher to have the students wash their hands or use wipes after handling food. If necessary, supply extra wipes for the teacher to have on hand for students to use if they eat foods that contain your child's allergen.

Easter

Here comes Peter Cottontail! Create your own family traditions with Easter basket substitutions. Instead of decorating allergenic hard-boiled eggs, buy wooden, plaster, or Styrofoam eggs and hop on down to your local craft store to purchase other fun items that you can paint and design yourself. Bubbles, seeds symbolizing springtime planting, pencils, erasers, themed books, gift cards, and small toys all make great basket fillers. Then add allergen-free candies and other joyful surprises.

Be advised that most Easter candy sold in grocery stores contains some of the Big 8: milk, eggs, peanuts, and tree nuts. It is pivotal to pay close attention to the "May Contain" portion on candy labels, as many list allergen ingredients that may have contaminated the product. Excellent allergy-free Easter candies are sold on the Web, so plan ahead as many need to be mail ordered in advance. Vermont Nut Free Chocolates has delicious seasonal, safe goodies, and Divvies many sweets are almost always free of all Big 8 allergens, so check their websites. Additionally, AllerGrocer .com has chocolate Easter bunnies and plenty of other holiday goodies.

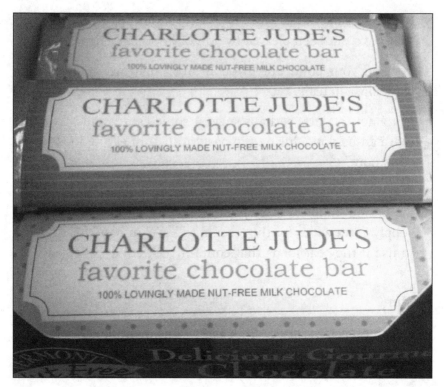

Allergy-safe chocolates from Vermont Nut Free Chocolate,
with handmade labels by the author.

Easter is an excellent holiday for make-your-own allergen-safe goodies. If you're feeling ambitious, you can have fun making your own Easter candy and treats from scratch. Candy molds can be purchased at local craft stores, with options ranging from chocolate eggs to lollipops, complete with sticks. Be sure to read ingredient labels carefully, and purchase allergen-safe dairy-free and nut-free chocolate chips. These can be melted down so they work just like Baker's chocolate; then pour or spoon the liquid chocolate into your fancy candy molds. Refrigerate for at least two hours until firm, and voila! For an over-the-top design element, you can decorate your candies with safe sprinkles and wrap them in festive papers or colorful plastic wrap before placing them artfully in an Easter basket.

Passover

The Passover holiday commemorates an important time in ancient Jewish history. It is celebrated in the home by holding a special ceremonial dinner, called a seder, when Jewish families read a holy text that includes eating traditional and symbolic foods. Advance planning for the eight days of Passover (Pesach) is a must.

Similar to Easter, Vermont Nut Free Chocolates offers a wide array of Passover-themed candies available for mail order. The traditional seder plate, however—the central part of the Passover table—includes a number of Big 8 food allergens. A simple yet appropriate substitution for a seder is wheat-free matzoh meal powder or whole matzos, which can be mail-ordered from several sites on the Internet. Traditional *Charoset* recipes contain allergenic walnuts and almonds, so pepitas (dry roasted pumpkin seeds) or even sunflower seeds and sesame seeds are appropriate substitutes. Two possible alternatives for the traditional roasted egg are a mushroom or even an edible flower. The mushroom is a closer visual analogy to an egg, but a flower is an apt symbol for spring and for rebirth. Both are great allergy-safe options.

Halloween

In 2011, I was asked by CNN and Yahoo! News to provide Halloween tips and suggestions. Here is the checklist I provided.

- Ask friends and neighbors that a separate bowl of allergen-free candy be made available. (Parents can also opt to distribute their own treats to neighbors before the trick-or-treating begins.)

- The concept of a decoy candy bag: Purchase two identical bags and fill one with a wide range of allergy-safe candies and, at the end of the evening, simply swap out the bag so the child has the adventure of going door-to-door with zero risk of a reaction.

- Older children can opt to trick-or-treat for charity, through organizations like UNICEF.

On our neighborhood block, I host an annual bash complete with a nut-free tent so there's a nice, big, safe zone for allergy sufferers. There's a fun sign I designed (complete with the Planter's Peanut in costume!), so every nut-allergic trick-or-treater for blocks can come in and indulge. We fill the tent with pounds and pounds of candy and toys, with wine for the adults, and make our own Haunted House zone where the festivity of the holiday can be celebrated to the fullest in a completely safe environment.

Thanksgiving, Channukah, and Christmas

Winter holidays offer special challenges for food-allergic folks. Here are ten tips to help you get through the holiday season safely and joyously.

Top Ten Party Tips for Food Allergies for the Winter Holiday Season

1. Hosts: Please keep food labels for everything used to prepare a festive homemade holiday meal so an allergic guest may double-check the ingredient list.

2. Hosts: If there's someone with a food allergy and guests want to contribute to the party, suggest flowers, wine, or holiday-themed napkins and plates instead of food items.

   Guests: Frey Vineyards in Mendocino, California, is historically America's first organic and biodynamic winery free of chemicals. Bringing your host a bottle of this wine is an elegant and affordable way to enhance the celebration; plus it's safe for people with sulfite allergies.

3. Don't overlook Tom Turkey! Some prebasted turkeys contain soy, wheat, and dairy. Instead look for turkeys labeled "Nat-

ural," which by law must be minimally processed. Some free-range, all-natural, fresh turkeys are free of antibiotics, hormones, and allergens. So ask for one!

4. Avoiding cross-contamination of utensils and surfaces when preparing foods is a must. Rinsing a knife that chopped walnuts is insufficient; thoroughly scrub all utensils and surfaces with soap and water and wipe clean. Even trace amounts of a food can cause a reaction for highly allergic people.

5. Ambitious home chefs: How about trying color-coded cooking utensils this year? A bright red silicone spatula or a nifty lime green serving spoon is sure to alert food-allergic guests. Many large box stores stock seasonal arrays of themed and brightly colored utensils a month or two in advance of the holiday season.

6. If a guest brings a food item that contains allergens, and there's an allergic diner at the table, you could accept it if it's well-sealed and donate it later to a friend or a soup kitchen. Some cities even have volunteer organizations dedicated to alleviating hunger. After a free phone call, their volunteers, who deliver more than 10 tons of food a week to agencies feeding people in need, will pick up a donation. In San Francisco, for example, a Google search turned up www.FoodRunners.org.

7. Guests: If you're allergic and flying to visit friends or family, make some simple allergy-free foods that travel well and ship them to your host's home a week or more in advance, so you're sure they'll arrive in time for your visit.

8. Guests: If your host has food allergies, you can always bring a gift of unpeeled fruit or a prepackaged seasonal safe food, with ingredient lists that your host says is A-OK.

9. Guests: If you're food allergic and even if the party you're invited to is not a potluck, why not offer to bring a safe dish or two so there's definitely something you can eat. Your host will be thankful not to have to prepare separate food items, and sharing dishes that are allergen-free will delight everyone there!

10. Guests: If you are allergic, always let your host or restaurant
    where you're celebrating know in advance—don't assume they
    will remember. Even a restaurant where you frequently dine
    may not immediately remember you and your medical con-
    dition at long holiday banquet tables with prix fixe meals. Be
    sure to remember to always bring your own medication and
    carry your grab-n-go medical bag *just in case of emergency.*

HOLIDAY STUFFINGS

Stuffing often contains various food allergens, and all these proteins
can become absorbed into the chicken, duck, or turkey during the cooking process. Ask the chef or host cook questions about all the stuffing
ingredients, and, if necessary, plan ahead: Make arrangements to bring
your own allergy-free stuffing or make sure the stuffing is cooked separately from the meat.

SPECIAL OCCASION CELEBRATIONS: BIRTHDAYS AND WEDDINGS

As equally festive—or even more so!—than a holiday celebration
is a milestone birthday party or even a life-changing wedding.

Birthdays

The highlight of each child's year is his or her birthday party celebrated alongside friends and family. However, food allergies in
children make it very difficult to find creative ways to celebrate
special events such as birthday parties. However, your child does
not have to feel different at his or her own birthday party. Stay
inventive and remember: Some great family rituals are experienced
together each year, and every new birthday is an opportunity to
make even more traditions.

Birthday Party Checklist

- Party bags and favors: Double-check at your party supply store to ensure any edibles are allergen-safe.

- Party venue: Bowling alleys and even pools sometimes have common food and beverage areas. Be certain to contact any rental facility well in advance to make sure it's able to safely accommodate you or your allergic child. When you find one, discuss your family's food allergy with the manager and devise a plan to meet your safety needs.

- Party piñata: Either check all prepared piñata candy prizes yourself or purchase an empty piñata that you can stuff with allergy-free candies and treats.

- Snacks and cake: If you are ordering snacks and cakes from a bakery, be certain to explain the food-allergy medical condition thoroughly. With a little planning, the birthday celebrant can eat everything at his or her own party.

- Attending a party as a guest: If you or your allergenic child are guests, attending a birthday party might mean having to skip the birthday cake and other treats. However, if you plan ahead and discuss it with the host, you can bring a decoy cake slice from home or a decoy cupcake that can be enjoyed safely with the rest of the gang. Until you're sure your child is in charge of his or her allergy, always remind him or her about food-allergy safety rules before attending a friend's party. These include not eating anything without clearing it through Mom and Dad and never sharing food from another guest's plate, no matter how tempting.

- Guests and gifts: Let guests know in advance, in writing or in an electronic invitation, that gifts for the birthday boy or girl must be allergen-safe.

- Don't focus your party on the food: At many birthday parties, food-allergic children who attend as guests are unable to eat most of the usual goodies, and they are, unfortunately, often resigned to passing on that cookie or yummy-looking cupcake. So for your own event, opt to not make food the focal point of the party. Instead, plan a fun theme such as a carnival or a skating party where the children will be busy playing games or skating rather than eating.

Weddings

When you or your future spouse have food allergies, you have a unique set of challenges: getting through all the hectic planning, your wedding ceremony and food-filled reception, and honeymoon all while staying sane and avoiding an allergic reaction. Catering companies and chefs are aces at handling special requests pertaining to food allergies. So book your caterer early—some happy couples plan a full year in advance—and make sure to explain your condition thoroughly before you arrange for menus and a tasting. Tastings are a festive bonding experience for you and your partner, and you may be able to have it in your own home. Once you have a menu for your big day, you can plan for your allergen-free wedding cake. Former U.S. President Bill Clinton's daughter, Chelsea, famously served wheat-free wedding cake—and wheat-free bread—at her nuptials. There are three basic options for a safe wedding cake.

1. A completely allergen-free tiered cake. If you have very few allergies and know of a competent, trustworthy bakery that makes allergy-free cakes, this might be an option. Note that it's best to do this only if you are positive that the bakery is allergy-aware, either through being a past customer or through word-of-mouth from friends. Yelp.com is a good way to evaluate local businesses in your area. Be extra careful since you do not want to have an allergic reaction on one of the most important days of your life!

2. A bride and groom allergen-free cake alongside a second bakery cake. If you have a lot of allergies or want your guests to have a conventional cake, you may want to choose this option. Speak to the bakery about how this would work and how they will avoid cross-contamination.

3. A homemade wedding cake, one that you and your partner bake yourselves, which is guaranteed to be free of your allergens! If you have lots of allergies, are afraid of cross-contamination, or simply don't trust or don't find a bakery to make a cake that is free of your allergens, you may want to make the cake or ask a trusted friend who loves to bake to make it—what a great wedding gift! Check your local library for food-allergy cookbooks with recipes that fit your allergen-free diet. Be sure to test-run a few of the recipes so you find the one that's perfect for your wedding.

Wedding Caterer Checklist

Are you getting married or planning a very special event that is going to be catered? First, congratulations! Depending on your budget, finding delicious and nutritious elegantly catered food may take a little exploration within your community. Finding a caterer who is able to adhere to your food-allergy requirements presents its own unique set of rules. Here are a few tips to enable you to have a successful—and safe—event:

• In your initial call or email to a prospective caterer, be certain to thoroughly explain your dietary restriction.

• Give the caterer a list of all your or your partner's food allergies in writing at your first meeting. At this time, openly discuss any concerns you have, including foods that have hidden ingredients.

• As you develop your dream menu, request a tasting and then be sure to reconfirm all ingredients before trying the dishes.

This will help you feel at ease—very important at your own wedding!—and ensure you like the taste of the food as well.

- Be sure to write your severe food allergy into your wedding day catering contract. Why not request a completely nut-free or milk-free prep kitchen for your once-in-a- lifetime special day?

- Follow up as your wedding gets closer to reconfirm your special details and food-allergy requirements.

- On your big day, make sure to take time to meet with the on-site catering staff to ensure your food-allergy requirements have been met.

- After your wedding, make sure to include your caterer in your thank-you-card list, since the firm played an integral role in making your magical day a safe and successful fairy tale!

9

Recipes

I t's time to celebrate healthy and fun cooking, and enjoy a plethora of ways to make healthy, special food for allergic friends and family (and nonallergic, too)! These recipes are allergen-free versions of many traditional favorites for everyone to enjoy. Baking without the standard ingredients might at first seem daunting to even the most seasoned home chef, but as we food-allergic folks are well aware: *Different foods can truly be better—because they are healthy and safe.* All these recipes are tried and true, and substitutions abound. The challenge of cooking and preparing particular meals with substitutions is particularly inspiring. Necessity is the mother of invention. And allergen-safe baking is deeply rewarding. It presents the opportunity for the ultimate in personal creative expression.

HOW TO MAKE ALLERGY SUBSTITUTIONS IN YOUR FAVORITE RECIPES

When you or a member of your family is diagnosed with a food allergy, there's absolutely no need to put away all those favorite cookbooks or pass by every recipe you come across that has allergens. At the same time, substituting certain culinary foods for allergy-safe cooking isn't just as simple as, say, replacing cow's milk with rice milk or all-purpose wheat flour with oat flour. That's because cooking is part science, and browning and baking create flavor and even change the color of our foods. So not every potential substitute ingredient—even if it seems similar in taste— works the same way in a recipe. Scientists describe the seven basic tastes as bitter, salty, sour, astringent, sweet, pungent, and savory. This is important when thinking about flavorful food-allergy substitutions in your home kitchen.

When shopping for ingredients, safe substitutes can be found in a number of places. You can typically find a good selection at your regular grocery store. For example, nondairy milk substitutes are widely available in most shops, and allergy-friendly cereals are starting to become easier to find in mainstream supermarkets. Even a dairy-free sour cream alternative exists: Tofutti's Sour Supreme. For eggs, you can purchase Ener-G's Egg Replacer, the best alternative on the market. To avoid eggs in mayonnaise, try buying the popular vegan alternative, Veganaise. Consider trying Seitan, which is a meat substitute made from wheat gluten, as a soy-free substitute for tofu. While its texture is not quite the same as tofu, both are equally high in protein and can be used like meat in stir-frys, soups, and chilis.

Wheat-free pasta has become increasingly available in the marketplace. The major options are made of rice, quinoa, beans, and those made from many grains, with rice pastas being the most common. All have slightly different textures and tastes, so which one you prefer is mostly a matter of your own personal preference. These pastas hold up well even in lasagnas and soups. Many of my friends recommend Bragg's Liquid Aminos as a tasty, unfermented, totally wheat-free substitute for soy sauce.

The closest peanut butter substitute available is Sunbutter, which is a sunflower seed butter made in a dedicated facility. There are also pumpkin seed butters and soy butters. If you live in a larger city that has a co-op or specialty food store, you can find many allergy-free foods there, and sometimes they even have their own aisle.

Here's a step-by-step guide to figuring out when substitutions may work and which potential substitutes will give you the best results.

1. Determine how major a role your allergen plays in the recipe. It's not possible to make a meringue without eggs, a gelato without cream, or a crusty Italian bread without wheat flour. You may still be able to make something approximating an allergen-free version of these classic dishes from a dietetic recipe, but substituting from a recipe involving eggs, dairy, or wheat is not likely to be successful because the chemistry of the substitutes will be so different.

2. If your allergen is a relatively minor part of the recipe, then analyze it roughly based on its component parts. For instance, egg whites are protein with a little bit of water, as are tofu and milk. Wheat flour is protein and starch. This analysis doesn't have to be exact by any means, but you do need to have a rough idea of whether the allergen in the recipe includes proteins, starches, or water to help you make an accurate substitution.

3. Figuring out the role the allergen plays in the recipe may require some guesswork, so here are a few rules of thumb to follow:

   • In a recipe with a batter, like fried chicken or tempura vegetables, flour is used on the outside to protect the vegetables, meat, or fish. Egg, milk, or buttermilk may be used to hold the batter on.

   • In a recipe with a sauce, it helps to know that flour, dairy products, or eggs may be used to thicken the sauce.

   • In a baked good, protein is used to help hold the baked structure together.

4. Find an appropriate substitute that has similar component parts and can play the same role in the recipe. The best substitutes are often similar to the ingredient in taste, composition, and texture. But this is not always the case. Because eggs and milk have similar components, it is sometimes possible to

replace the dairy in a baked good by adding extra eggs and water. And sometimes when wheat is being used more for its protein than for its starch, high-protein bean flour makes a better substitute than rice flour, even though bean flour has a much stronger taste.

Basic Allergen Substitutes for Recipes

A range of products can easily be substituted for milk, eggs, wheat, and peanuts and tree nuts in many recipes. Try out the following ingredients in your favorite recipes until you find a substitution that suits your taste buds.

Substitutions for Milk

- Grated Brazil nuts instead of *grated parmesan cheese*
- Crumbled tofu instead of *ricotta cheese*
- Unsweetened coconut cream instead of *heavy cream*
- Soy, rice, coconut, or almond milk instead of *milk*
- Vegetable or chicken stock in a soup or sauce instead of *milk*

Substitutions for Eggs

- Tahini sauce instead of *mayonnaise*
- Mashed banana in a cake recipe instead of *eggs*
- Cooked chicken or tofu instead of *hard-boiled egg*

Substitutions for Wheat

- Lettuce leaves to wrap sandwiches instead of *bread*
- Almond meal for baking cakes and breads instead of *flour*
- Coarsely ground almonds or other nut instead of *bread crumbs*
- Shaved carrots, spaghetti squash, or zucchini instead of *pasta*

Substitutions for Peanuts and Tree Nuts

- Sunflower or pumpkin seeds instead of *peanuts and tree nuts*

- Finely chopped red onion or diced celery for a *nutty, crunchy garnish*

- Pan-fried chickpeas or other canned beans instead of *pine nuts*

MAIN MEALS

Here are recipes for a few classic meals that I've acquired over the years. May they inspire you to devise your own recipes that suit your family's lifestyle and palate.

• • • • • • • • • • • • •

Allergen-Free Barbecued Lamb Kebabs

Serves 4 • Prep time: 2 hours • Cook time: 8–10 minutes

Marinated lamb cubes

3/4 cup olive oil

2/3 cup fresh lemon juice

6 large garlic cloves, minced

2 tablespoons chopped fresh mint

4 teaspoons grated lemon peel

2 teaspoons ground black pepper

2 teaspoons ground coriander

1 teaspoon ground cumin

4 teaspoons salt

4 pounds well-trimmed boneless leg of lamb
cut into 2-inch cubes

Vegetables for kebabs

4 red onions, each cut into 8 chunks

1 red pepper, seeded, cut into chunks

1 orange pepper, seeded, cut into chunks

16 10-inch bamboo skewers, soaked in water overnight,
if possible, so they don't burn

1. Whisk olive oil, lemon juice, all herbs, spices, and salt together in medium bowl to blend marinade.

2. Add lamb to marinade; toss to coat. Marinate 2 hours at room temperature or cover and refrigerate overnight.

3. Prepare barbecue at medium-high heat.

4. Remove lamb from marinade.

5. Thread lamb cubes and vegetable chunks alternately onto skewers, dividing equally.

6. Grill lamb to desired doneness, turning occasionally, about 8 minutes for medium rare.

Serve skewers over rice or as desired. Enjoy!

· · · · · · · · · · · · ·

Allergen-Free Holiday Eve Prime Ribs and Gravy

*Season's eatings for each and every allergic guest;
free of all Big 8 allergens.*

*Prep time: 10 minutes • Cook time: 45–60 minutes
depending on size of roast*

1 standing rib roast with bones cut away and tied
(ask your butcher to prepare)

Salt and pepper to taste

1. Ask your butcher for 3–7 ribs; estimate serving is two people per rib.

2. Take roast out of refrigerator and unwrap. Roast 3 hours before cooking; roast should be brought to room temperature before entering the oven.

3. Preheat oven to 500°F.

4. Generously sprinkle salt and pepper over entire roast.

5. Place roast fat side up, rib side down in a roasting pan in the oven. Insert meat thermometer into thickest part of the roast.

6. After 15 minutes, reduce heat to 325°F. Allow 13–15 minutes per pound for rare meat and 15–17 minutes per pound for medium.

7. Roast until internal temperature on the meat thermometer registers 115°F for rare or 125°F for medium.

8. Remove from the oven and let roast rest for 20 minutes, loosely covered with foil prior to carving.

9. With kitchen scissors, cut the strings and remove the bones.

With a sharp knife, slice meat against the grain and serve.

Prime Rib Gravy

1. Place roasting pan with drippings directly on stove at medium heat.

2. Whisk 1 tablespoon cornstarch and slowly add water until gravy is smooth. Season with salt, pepper, and desired herbs.

Pour generously over meat or into a gravy boat so guests can serve themselves.

WHEAT-FREE HOLIDAY GRAVIES

Marinades and soy sauce, broth and bouillon may use wheat as flavors and seasonings. Always avoid a seasoning or gravy packet. To thicken gravy, whisk in a tablespoon of sweet rice flour, potato flour, or an arrowroot starch slurry.

• • • • • • • • • • •

Classic Homemade
Wheat-Free Pizza Recipe

*Bob's Red Mill Gluten-Free All-Purpose Baking Flour is
a good substitute for wheat. It contains garbanzo flour,
potato starch, tapioca flour, sorghum flour, and fava flour.
Note: It is manufactured in a facility that
also uses tree nuts and soy.*

*Makes 2 quarts dough for two 10- to-12-inch pizzas, which serve 2–4.
Prep time: 2 hours • Cook time: 30 minutes*

Wheat-Free Pizza Dough

1^1/$_2$ cups warm water

1 package of active dry yeast

2 tablespoons extra virgin olive oil

3 ^{1}/$_2$ cups Bob's Red Mill Gluten-Free
All-Purpose Baking Flour

2 teaspoons salt

1 teaspoon sugar

Pizza Topping

Extra virgin olive oil

Cornmeal

28-ounce can of plum tomato purée

Garlic cloves, thinly sliced

Mozzarella and parmigiano-reggiano cheese, shredded

Pepperoni, thinly sliced (optional)

Mushrooms, thinly sliced (optional)

Pesto or "Pistou" sauce (optional; see page 111)

1. In large electric mixer bowl, combine warm water and yeast. Stir to dissolve completely and let mixture rest for 5 minutes.

2. Mix in olive oil, baking flour, salt, and sugar on low speed with mixing paddle attachment for 60 seconds. Replace paddle with dough hook attachment and knead for 8 minutes until dough is elastic and smooth. (Note: You can mix and knead by hand if you don't have a mixer. However, if your hand-mixed dough is not elastic and smooth, slowly add additional baking flour a little at a time.)

3. Remove dough ball from mixing bowl and coat lightly with extra virgin olive oil.

4. Cover with plastic wrap in a bowl and place dough in a warm place for $1^1/_2$ hours to rise.

5. Preheat oven to 450°F.

6. Remove plastic wrap and punch the dough down. Then divide the dough in half and hand-form two round balls of dough.

7. Place each in its own bowl, cover with plastic wrap, and let sit for 10 additional minutes.

8. Take each ball of dough and flatten it with your hands on a floured surface. Use your fingertips to press the dough until each reaches the desired diameter—10 to 12 inches. Use your palm to flatten the edge of the dough where it is thicker. Then pinch the edge to form the crust.

9. Brush the tops of the dough with olive oil.

10. Lightly sprinkle flat pizza baking sheets or pizza stones with cornmeal, and place dough on them.

11. Spoon on tomato sauce purée, top with thinly sliced garlic to taste, then sprinkle with cheese, and place optional desired toppings on top.

12. Bake pizzas one at a time until the crust is browned, 10–12 minutes.

Cheese will be hot. Cool as desired and serve.

• • • • • • • • • • • •

Allergen-Free Herbed Mashed Potatoes

Who doesn't enjoy a rich, creamy dairy-free accompaniment to a rib roast?

Makes 8–10 servings • Prep time: 15 minutes • Cook time: 20 minutes

2 pounds Yukon Gold potatoes

2–4 cloves garlic, peeled

1 cup rice milk (not vanilla)

2 tablespoons olive oil

1 tablespoon chopped fresh parsley

Salt and pepper to taste

1. Bring a large pot of water to a boil.

2. Wash potatoes and chop them roughly into quarters and add to boiling water. Toss in garlic cloves. When potatoes are soft when pierced with a fork, remove from heat, drain thoroughly, and return potatoes and garlic to pot.

3. Pour rice milk and olive oil into pot, and mash with hand-held potato masher. Add parsley, salt, and pepper to taste.

Scoop mashed potatoes into a serving bowl and serve hot.

SAUCES

You can use a variety of allergen-free sauces to safely spice up your meals. All of these can be used indefinitely as long as they are refrigerated.

•   •   •   •   •   •   •   •   •   •   •   •   •   •   •   •

Peanut-Free and Tree Nut–Free Pesto or Pistou Sauce

Pistou is an olive oil–based basil sauce from the south of France that closely resembles Italian pesto, but without the nuts. Like its Italian cousin, Pistou can also be served atop pizza, tossed with pasta, spread over toasted baguette slices, or as an accompaniment to grilled meats, poultry, fish, and vegetables.

Prep time: 10 minutes • No cook time

2 cloves garlic

3 cups fresh basil leaves

$1/2$ cup fresh grated parmesan cheese

$1/2$ cup olive oil

Squeeze of lemon to taste

Salt and pepper to taste

1. In a food processor or blender, chop the garlic until it is minced.

2. Add basil and cheese, and start to blend. Slowly drizzle in olive oil while machine is running, and blend until smooth.

3. Squeeze in lemon juice to taste, and add salt and pepper to taste.

Serve immediately, or store in airtight glass container and/or freeze. Shake well before use.

Classic Egg-Free and Fish-Free Caesar Salad Dressing

Serves 2–4 portions • Prep time: 10 minutes • No cook time

1 clove garlic, finely chopped

Juice of 1 lemon

1 teaspoon hot sauce (We adore Tabasco brand.)

1 teaspoon fish-free Worcestershire sauce (see page 112)

1 teaspoon Dijon mustard

1/3 cup extra virgin olive oil

1 cup shredded parmesan cheese

Salt and pepper to taste

1. Whisk all ingredients by hand or in a blender.
Serve tossed well on salads.

Homemade Fish-Free Worcestershire Sauce

Prep time: 20 minutes • Cook time: 35 minutes •
Storage time: 30 days

1 yellow onion, chopped

2 cloves garlic

1 1/2-inch-thick slice ginger

3 tablespoons dried mustard seed

1 teaspoon whole black peppercorns

2 teaspoons crushed red pepper flakes

1 cinnamon stick

1 teaspoon whole cloves

2 cups cider vinegar

$1/2$ cup dark molasses

$1/2$ cup soy-free soy sauce (see page 114)

$1^1/_2$ tablespoons sea salt

$1/2$ teaspoon curry powder

15 pitted kalamata olives

1 cup water

1. Purchase cooking cheesecloth and baker's twine.

2. Make a bundle of onion, garlic, ginger, mustard seeds, peppercorns, red pepper flakes, and cinnamon stick, and tie off the bag.

3. In a large saucepan, combine your spice bag with vinegar, molasses, and soy sauce. Bring to a boil, reduce heat, and simmer for 30 minutes.

4. In a small bowl, combine salt, curry powder, and kalamata olives with water.

5. Add the salt combination to the saucepan and simmer for another 5 minutes.

6. Remove from heat, and pour the contents of saucepan, including spice bundle, into a quart jar. Seal and cover securely.

7. Place sealed jar in refrigerator for 30 days, shaking occasionally.

8. After one month, open jar and carefully strain just the liquid. Squeeze the spice bag over the strainer, then discard the bundle.

9. Bottle your sauce.

Keep refrigerated and shake well before use.

• • • • • • • • • • •

Soy-Free Homemade Soy Sauce

Prep time: 10 minutes • Cook time: 1 hour

2 cups low-sodium beef broth

2 teaspoons cider vinegar

1 teaspoon dark molasses

$1/8$ teaspoon ground ginger

Onion powder to taste

Garlic powder to taste

White pepper to taste

1. Combine all ingredients in a small saucepan, and boil uncovered until reduced to $1/2$ cup.

2. Remove from heat, cool, and pour contents of saucepan into a quart jar. Seal and cover securely.

Keep refrigerated and shake well before use.

BREAD, MUFFINS, BISCUITS, AND GRANOLA BARS

Everybody loves all kinds of breadstuffs, so here are allergen-free recipes that address specific needs. Feel free to experiment with these recipes to come up with variations that suit your palate.

● ● ● ● ● ● ● ● ● ● ● ● ● ●

Charlotte Jude's Favorite Peanut-Free and Tree Nut–Free Zucchini Bread

*Makes 2 loaves • Prep time: 15 minutes •
Cook time: 50–60 minutes*

3 eggs

1 cup vegetable oil

2 cups granulated sugar

2 cups grated zucchini (2 to 3 small zucchini)

2 teaspoons vanilla

3 cups all-purpose flour

1 teaspoon salt

1 teaspoon baking soda

1 teaspoon baking powder

1 tablespoon ground cinnamon

1. Beat eggs until light and foamy; add vegetable oil, sugar, zucchini, and vanilla.

2. Mix lightly with wisk or by hand, but blend thoroughly.

3. In separate bowl, lightly mix together flour, salt, baking soda, baking powder, and cinnamon.

4. Add dry ingredients to the egg mixture, stirring to blend.

5. Pour batter into two 9 x 5 x 3-inch loaf pans.

6. Preheat oven at 325°F.

6. Bake for 50 to 60 minutes, until a toothpick inserted near center of a loaf comes out clean.

Cool and serve.

• • • • • • • • • • • • • • • • • • • •

Allergen-Free Chewy Granola Bars

Prep time: 10 minutes • Cook time: 30 minutes

2 cups old-fashioned rolled oats (Quaker brand is good)

1 cup raw, chopped pumpkin seeds

$1/2$ cup raw, chopped sunflower seeds

1 cup honey

2 tablespoons butter

1 tablespoon vanilla extract

1 cup chopped dried fruit: cranberries, cherries, golden raisins,

california or mediterranean apricots

1 teaspoon salt

$1/4$ cup flax seeds

$1/4$ teaspoon cinnamon

$1/4$ cup allergy-free chocolate chips

1. Preheat the oven to 300°F.

2. Spread the oats, pumpkin seeds, and sunflower seeds on an ungreased cookie sheet and toast for 15 minutes until fragrant and browned.

3. In a saucepan, combine the honey and butter over medium heat, and add vanilla extract.

4. Grease a 9 x 13-inch glass baking dish.

5. Adjust oven to 350°F.

6. Combine the dry oat and wet butter mixtures in a mixing bowl. Add dried fruit and salt. Blend well and sprinkle with flax seeds and cinnamon.

7. Press into the prepared baking dish.

8. Add chocolate chips, pressing them into the top of the oat mixture.

9. Cook for 30 minutes or until the granola starts to brown on the edges.

Cool completely and cut into large squares. Store in an airtight container.

* * * * * * * * * * * * * * *

Peanut-Free, Tree Nut–Free, Dairy-Free, Egg-Free Dinner Biscuits

Makes 8 biscuits • Prep time: 10 minutes • Cook time: 15–20 minutes

1 cup all-purpose flour

1 tablespoon baking powder

1 teaspoon granulated sugar

$1/2$ teaspoon salt

1 cup rice or soy milk

2 tablespoons light nondairy spread, melted for brushing

1. Preheat oven to 425°F and line a baking sheet with parchment paper. Set aside.

2. In a medium bowl, whisk together the flour, baking powder, sugar, and salt. Add the rice or soy milk slowly, stirring with a rubber spatula until the dough just comes together yet isn't sticky.

3. Turn onto a lightly floured surface and knead until dough is soft and smooth.

4. Pat the dough into a circle about $1/2$ inch thick. Use a 2-inch biscuit cutter to make eight rounds, reshaping the dough as necessary.

5. Brush the top of each biscuit with melted nondairy spread, and bake for 15–20 minutes or until very light golden brown.

Cool and serve.

• • • • • • • • • • • • • • • • • • •

Peanut-Free, Tree Nut–Free, Egg-Free, Milk-Free "Berry Delicious" Blueberry Muffins

Makes 12 muffins • Prep time: 15 minutes •
Cook time: 28–30 minutes

2 cups all-purpose flour

$3/4$ teaspoon baking soda

$1/2$ teaspoon salt

1 cup sugar

1 cup soy milk

$1/3$ cup canola oil

1 tablespoon white vinegar

1 cup fresh or frozen blueberries

1. Preheat oven to 350°F.

2. Grease muffin pan with nonstick baking spray or use cupcake/muffin cups.

3. Whisk flour, baking soda, and salt in a medium mixing bowl. Set aside.

4. In a large separate mixing bowl, mix sugar, soy milk, oil, and vinegar until smooth and foamy.

5. Add the dry ingredients to the wet ingredients and blend well.

6. Fill the muffin tins with batter, approximately 2 tablespoons for each muffin.

7. Distribute blueberries gently into each muffin tin until they are enveloped with batter.

8. Bake the muffins for 28 to 30 minutes.

Cool and serve.

DESSERTS AND SWEET TREATS

Allergen-free ice cream and cake are essential for birthday parties and other family occasions, and risk-free pumpkin pie is needed to complete Thanksgiving and end-of-year holiday meals. Sweet treats are always fun for movie viewing either in a theater or in your home.

Allergen-Free Vanilla Cake Frosting

Prep time: 10 minutes

2 pounds confectioners sugar

1 cup shortening

2 teaspoons vanilla

Dash of salt

8 tablespoons water

1. Place confectioners sugar in the mixing bowl of an electric mixer.

2. Chop shortening into small chunks, and place on top of the powdered sugar.

3. Add vanilla and salt and mix.

4. Add the water 1 tablespoon at a time evenly into the mixture using the mixer.

5. Blend together until well combined and frosting is light and fluffy.

Frost cake and serve.

. . . .

Milk-Free and Egg-Free Homemade Vanilla Ice Cream

Serves 4 • Prep time: 10 minutes • Cook time: 30–40 minutes •
Freezer time: 3 hours

$1^1/_2$ cups soy milk powder

$3^1/_2$ cups soy milk

$^2/_3$ cup water

$1^1/_2$ cups sugar

1 tablespoon vanilla

1 teaspoon apple cider vinegar

1 pinch of kosher salt

1. In a blender, combine the soy milk powder, soy milk, pinch of kosher salt, and water until blended.

2. Combine the soy milk mixture with the sugar, vanilla, and vinegar in a small saucepan over medium-low heat.

3. Cook for 30–40 minutes, stirring constantly until the mixture is thick and syrupy in consistency.

4. Pour the mixture into a 9 x 5-inch metal loaf pan and freeze uncovered for 1 hour.

5. Remove pan from the freezer, and scrape the mixture into a blender.

6. Blend on high for 30 seconds.

7. Place the mixture back in the pan and into the freezer, uncovered.

8. Now here's the trick: Repeat twice (every 30 minutes during the next hour), so ice cream will be creamy and not crunchy with ice crystals.

9. Place the mixture back in the pan, cover, and freeze for final hour before serving.

Serve ice cold, with desired toppings.

Peanut-Free, Tree Nut–Free, Dairy-Free, Egg-Free Double Chocolate Cake

A traditional cake includes egg and milk products.
Enjoy this delicious alternative!

Makes 8 servings • Prep time: 15 minutes •
Cook time: 30–35 minutes

1$^1/_2$ cups all-purpose flour

$^1/_2$ teaspoon salt

1 cup white sugar

$^1/_3$ cup unsweetened cocoa powder

1 teaspoon baking soda

5 tablespoons vegetable oil

1 tablespoon white vinegar

1 teaspoon vanilla extract

1 cup cold water

$^1/_2$ cup semisweet, dairy-free chocolate chips

1. Preheat oven to 350°F. Grease an 8 x 8-inch baking pan.

2. In a large bowl, combine flour, salt, sugar, cocoa powder, and baking soda, and mix well.

3. Add oil, vinegar, and vanilla extract to dry ingredients, and stir well.

4. Add cold water and stir until batter is smooth. Stir in chocolate chips, and pour batter into greased pan.

5. Bake for 30 to 35 minutes, until a toothpick inserted in center comes out clean.

Cool on a rack and serve.

• •

Allergen-Free Holiday Pumpkin Pie

Makes 8 servings • Prep time: 20 minutes • Cook time: 1 hour

Crust

$1\frac{1}{2}$ cups Bob's Red Mill Gluten-Free All-Purpose Baking Flour

1 teaspoon salt

$\frac{1}{2}$ cup vegetable oil

2 tablespoons French vanilla rice creamer

Pie Filling

2 cups canned pumpkin

1 cup French vanilla rice creamer

$\frac{3}{4}$ cup brown sugar

$\frac{1}{4}$ cup cornstarch

1 tablespoon dark corn syrup

1 teaspoon ground cinnamon

$\frac{1}{8}$ teaspoon ground ginger

$\frac{1}{2}$ teaspoon ground nutmeg

$\frac{1}{2}$ teaspoon salt

$\frac{1}{8}$ teaspoon ground cloves

1. Preheat the oven to 425°F.

2. Stir together flour and salt.

3. In a separate bowl, whisk together the vegetable oil and rice creamer until creamy.

4. Pour oil mixture into flour mixture, and mix well until blended.

5. Pat the crust into bottom and sides of a 9-inch greased pie pan.

6. Bake for 15 minutes. Remove and set aside.

7. Decrease oven to 350°F.

8. Meanwhile, place all pie filling ingredients in a blender, and blend until combined, approximately 30 seconds.

• • • • • • • • • • • •

Allergen-Free Brownies

Makes 20 servings • Prep time: 10 minutes •
Cook time: 20–25 minutes

1 cup potato flour

1 cup brown rice flour

2 cups white sugar

$^1/_2$ cup unsweetened cocoa powder

$^1/_2$ teaspoon baking soda

$^5/_8$ teaspoon cream of tartar

$1^1/_2$ teaspoons sea salt

3 overripe bananas, mashed

$1^1/_2$ cups vegetable oil

1. Preheat the oven to 325°F.

2. Grease a 9 x13-inch glass baking dish.

3. In a large bowl, mix together the potato flour, rice flour, sugar, cocoa powder, baking soda, cream of tartar, and salt.

4. Blend together the mashed bananas and oil in a separate bowl.

5. Stir the banana mixture into the dry ingredients until well blended.

6. Spread evenly in the bottom of the prepared pan.

7. Bake 20 to 25 minutes, until the brownies appear dry on the top. Do not overbake. Cool completely, cut into squares, and serve.

9. Pour the pie filling into the piecrust. Place foil around the edges of the crust, and bake for 60 minutes or until a knife inserted 1 inch from the crust comes out clean.

Cool pie on counter for 2 hours, and refrigerate overnight before serving.

* * * * * * * * * * * * *

Allergen-Free Movie Theater Caramel Corn

Be sure to eat it all up because it goes gooey quite quickly.

Serves 6 • Prep time: 30 minutes • Cook time: 1 hour

6 quarts plain popped popcorn

2 cups brown sugar

$1/2$ cup light corn syrup

1 cup nondairy spread

1 teaspoon salt

$1/2$ teaspoon baking soda

1 teaspoon vanilla extract

1. Preheat the oven to 250°F.

2. Place popcorn into two shallow greased baking pans.

3. Combine brown sugar, corn syrup, nondairy spread, and salt in a saucepan. Bring to a boil over medium heat, and stir frequently for 5 minutes.

4. Remove from the heat, and stir in baking soda and vanilla.

5. Pour immediately over popcorn, and stir to coat.

6. Bake 1 hour, stirring with spatula once after 30 minutes.

7. Turn out caramel corn on wax paper or nonstick baking sheet, and separate kernels.

Cool until room temperature and serve.

* * * * * * * * * * * * * * * *

Peanut-Free and Tree Nut–Free Charlotte Jude's Sunflower Butter Cups

Makes 12 treats • Prep time: 15 minutes •
Freezer time: 15 minutes

Mini muffin tin

Candy papers from a baking or craft store

12-ounce bag of allergen-free chocolate chips

12 teaspoons sunflower seed butter

1. Line mini muffin tin with candy papers.

2. Place chocolate chips in a heat-safe bowl and microwave for 30 seconds. Stir until smooth or repeat, if necessary.

3. Pour 1 tablespoon of melted chocolate into each candy paper.

4. Add 1 teaspoon of sunflower seed butter to center of each cup.

5. Top each cup with 1 tablespoon chocolate.

6. Place mini muffin tin in freezer to set for 15 minutes.

Serve cool or cold.

SCHOOL LUNCH-BOX RECIPES

Recipes for allergen-free school lunches are essential. Here are three substitutions. But with a little thought and practice, I'm confident you can create other recipes your child will safely enjoy.

• **Instead of a tuna fish sandwich, try:** Chicken salad sandwich on a bagel. With diced chicken, mix diced celery, diced apples, cut grapes, or dried cranberries, egg-free mayonnaise, a squeeze of lemon, and salt and pepper to taste.

- **Instead of a peanut butter and jelly sandwich, instead try:** Sunflower seed, soy, almond, or another safe butter with fresh fruit slices on allergy-safe bread.

- **Instead of a turkey and cheese wrap sandwich, try:** La Tortilla Factory offers wheat-free tortillas made with *teff* (an African grain). Spread tortilla with honey mustard, and stuff with turkey slices, dairy-free shredded cheese, sliced tomato, sliced cucumber, and lettuce leaves. Roll like a burrito.

Pack that thermos or cooler with allergy-free, high-protein brain food.

- Hummus topped with cucumbers and fresh vegetables

- Tortillas and mashed beans topped with shredded nondairy cheese

- Black bean burgers and avocado slices on a wheat-free bun

- Cooked brown rice with mild black bean salsa

- Homemade meatballs and marinara sauce

- Nondairy yogurt with fresh fruit slices

- Fruit smoothie

- Fresh fruit kebabs with dairy-free yogurt dipping sauce

- Fresh vegetable kebabs with salad dressing dip

- Rice or soy milk boxes

- Nut-free and/or wheat-free granola bars

- Roasted pumpkin and/or sunflower seeds

- Dried fruit

10

Go Live Your Life!

Food allergies affect people of all ages and income levels and families of all sizes. Finding the balance between remaining vigilant yet enjoying your life takes practice. Your life depends on a food-allergy action plan, yes, but your life also depends on the quality and enjoyment of each moment. The more you allow yourself to relax, the better you actually protect your health. There is a wide range of voices in our food-allergy world. Here are a few who asked to share:

As a woman, mother, and friend, I never thought allergies would affect my family until I found myself barely breathing after eating a certain shellfish. Severe allergies happened to others, not to me and my family. We ate organic, exercised, took really good care of ourselves, didn't get sick, and were never incapacitated by the "nut" allergies that affected so many of my friends. Until I learned that not only was I allergic to certain foods, my son was, too. For me, as an adult, I just knew to stay away from foods that didn't agree with me; for a young boy, allergies affected his everyday life. They affected how he did in school and how he interacted with others, and they altered the state of his everyday life. Allergies can take over a person's life in ways that many would never understand. It can be daunting, scary, and frustrating for all involved. Mireille Schwartz took my hand and offered an opportunity to feel normal, live a normal life, and bring balance to our home. We live with allergies, but now we manage them in a way that works for us. I hope this book will do for your family what Mireille did for mine. I am grateful.

Claudia Castillo Ross
Layfayette, California

We discovered our child had multiple allergies to soy, wheat, dairy, and sesame seeds, and the diagnosis was brutal. Everything scared us, and most of the time we didn't know what was going to happen next. We begged out of birthday parties and even skipped our annual family reunion in the Grand Canyon. Little by little, we got braver, but it took time. With help, we gradually got our lives back. Nothing is the same as it was, but we have found a way to still have fun and do normal stuff.

—J. Walsh, Philadelphia, Pennsylvania

Of course, being a preteen with a food allergy is hard, and only after a while did I start to adapt. Of course, it's never just gonna be "simple" or "easy." Life never is, but I know how to get by. My mother taught me that you always need to read labels and look out for cross-contamination and shared equipment, so I always look for "MAY CONTAIN PEANUTS AND TREE NUTS." After a while, it's gotten easier living with food allergies. Even my school has made the whole environment "no nuts!" Living with food allergies may be hard, but, with support and your smarts, it's not impossible.

—Bianca, Bay Area, California

"From my classroom it looks as if food-allergy survival fosters a peculiar outlook in an individual: This young person has learned at an early age how to be acutely sensitive to material conditions. Such youth know that what each human being has in common with every other is the necessity of coping with circumstance. That's an ancient point of view: you can find it in Hippocrates. When we meet young people with food allergies for the first time, we already know they've got something to contend with that's not of their own choosing. Starting from a private predicament, since we either share food or we don't, it doesn't take a great leap of the imagination for a young food-allergic person to grasp that everybody else in the world has troubles of a worldly kind, too. This material sensitivity gives a practical cast to the food-allergic person's way of feeling (and not feeling) empathy. It can also make our indifference to these allergies seem uniquely cruel. Yet such empathy contains within itself the origin of an openness and rationality that's going to become a lot more common pretty soon. The outcome is what you might call the terms of discourse: new ways of speaking and writing about food allergies. The rest will take care of itself."

—George N., private school teacher, 16 years in the classroom

When faced with food-allergy challenges, do your best to neutralize anxiety, as this fortifies your immune system. Diagnosis is only the first step on the path of learning to cope with food allergies. It takes time to integrate allergies into your life and adjust to your new "normal." While it doesn't seem possible at first, pretty soon living with your or your family member's food allergies will indeed become normal to you. It is absolutely possible to live a full, active life with food allergies, despite the stress and uncertainty that allergies can initially cause.

A 2008 review published in *Lancet* medical journal found there are four basic strategies that help individuals mentally adjust to a chronic illness, such as food allergy, and have happier, better health outcomes:

• **Exercise:** Regular physical activity can improve your mood and make you healthier—which then cycles around and improves your mood. Exercise won't change your food allergies, but it can reduce the physical impact of stress on your body.

- **Express your emotions:** Talking or writing about your feelings about your allergies and their impact on your life—both positive and negative—can actually make you physically healthier. Struggling to deal with everything yourself can make you feel isolated and increase your stress level.

- **Manage your allergies:** Learning to avoid your trigger foods and stick to your special diet can help you stay healthy. It can also help you be happier overall and better able to cope with the stress of living with allergies. When you feel confident that you can read labels, navigate a restaurant menu, or plan a vacation around your allergy, the feeling of success creates a background "buzz" of happiness that helps motivate you to keep on keeping yourself healthy.

- **Focus on the potential positive outcomes of your allergies:** Thinking about positive aspects of your food allergies such as eating healthier foods or having a renewed appreciation of life can help reduce your stress and lead to better health. Remind yourself of the good foods that you are able to eat, new friends you have made because of your food allergy, and other silver linings to your food-allergy cloud.[1]

Keep in mind the many reasons for optimism on the food-allergy front: There have been tremendous advances in medicine, education, and research over the last few years. Awareness is at an all-time high, with widespread comprehension that food allergy is a true disease and not "hysteria." In my lifetime I've had the distinct privilege of participating in the remarkable evolution of understanding food allergy better. To date, clinical trials at Mt. Sinai Hospital in New York City are currently unlocking a "cure" for egg allergy, and the day will come when scientists solve the riddle of this biological mystery.

Celebrate your friendships, celebrate your accomplishments! You and your family are doing your best with a challenging medical condition, and sometimes it takes courage to get out there and mingle with the crowd, board that airplane, take that plunge. Honestly, at times your food allergy is isolating, at times terrifying. Wherever you are along the food-allergy path—whether researching signs and symptoms, newly diagnosed, still struggling to learn to read food labels, or fully adapted to your new reality—it helps to recognize that you are on a journey. Yet here you are another year wiser and an integral part of the meeting at work, eating at the nightly dinner table, and enjoying the family vacation. So take a deep breath, bring your rescue meds, and live every day of your life to the fullest—full of adventures and new experiences. You deserve it.

Endnotes

Chapter 2

1. Justin M. Skripak, et al. "The natural history of IgE-mediated cow's milk allergy." *Journal of Allergy and Clinical Immunology.* Vol. 120 (November 2007): 1172–1177.

2. S. H. Sicherer, A. Muñoz-Furlong, H. A. Sampson. "Prevalence of seafood allergy in the United States determined by a random telephone survey." *Journal of Allergy and Clinical Immunology.* Vol. 113 (February 2004): S100.

Chapter 5

1. A. Nowak-Wegrzyn, M. K. Conover-Walker, R. A. Wood. "Food-allergic reactions in schools and preschools." *Archives of Pediatric and Adolescent Medicine.* Vol. 7 (July 2001): 790–795.

2. T. T. Perry, et al. "Distribution of peanut allergen in the environment." *Clinical Immunology.* Vol. 113 (May 2004): 803–1010.

Chapter 10

1. Dr. Denise de Ridder, et al. "Psychological adjustment to chronic disease." *The Lancet.* Vol. 372 (July 2008): 246–255.

Glossary

Note that terms defined in the Glossary are italicized when they appear in another definition.

Allergen: A food or substance that triggers an allergic reaction.

Allergenic: A food or substance that has the properties to trigger an allergic reaction.

Allergic Rhinitis: Commonly referred to as hay fever. The inflammation of the nasal passages caused by an allergic reaction to airborne substances.

Allergist: A doctor who specializes in the diagnosis, immunology, and treatment of allergies.

Anaphylaxis: An immediate, severe allergic reaction that causes difficulty breathing, swelling of the throat and tongue, and respiratory failure or shock due to a sudden drop in blood pressure. In extreme cases, it is sometimes fatal.

Angioedema: Swelling that typically accompanies *hives* and can occur anywhere in the body.

Antihistamine: Medication used to block the effects of *histamine*, the chemical released during an allergic reaction. It does not stop the reaction but prevents the reaction from triggering some symptoms. It is available as both a prescription and an over-the-counter medication.

Asthma: A medical condition that causes narrowing of the small airways in the lungs, often arising from an allergic reaction. Symptoms include wheezing, coughing, chest tightness, and shortness of breath.

Atopic: A state that makes people more likely to develop allergic reactions of any type. A hereditary, genetic predisposition.

Atopic dermatitis: A skin condition; itchy *eczema* caused or made worse by an allergic condition.

Auto injector: Device that enables food-allergic individuals to inject themselves with a premeasured dose of *epinephrine* medication. It is available by prescription as EpiPen® or Twinject®, and now as Auvi-Q™, a battery-powered, compact epinephrine device that talks a user through the step-by-step injection process.

Avoidance: A food regimen designed to assist food-allergic individuals who must steer clear of any product that triggers reactions.

Benadryl® (diphendydramine): A widely used *antihistamine* available in liquid, pill, or fastmelt/meltaway form. Very effective medication in treating food-allergy reactions, but in the event of a severe allergic reaction Benadryl® may not be completely effective, and *epinephrine* is required.

Biphasic allergic reaction: A second allergic reaction that occurs 2 to 6 hours after the first, often when the first wave of symptoms is under control.

Blind test: A *food-allergy* treatment study in which researchers know who is receiving treatment and who is not, but the patients do not.

Casien (and casienate): A milk *protein*. Present in all *dairy* products.

Cross-contamination: This occurs when one food comes in contact with another food and their *proteins* mix, which is often invisible to the eye. Usually occurs when a safe food is manufactured on the same equipment as an unsafe food or when safe food is prepared or served with tainted utensils. Each food then contains small trace particles of the other food, which can trigger an allergic response.

Dairy: Containing or made from cow's milk, which is one of the most common allergenic foods.

Dedicated facility: A manufacturing facility that is free from a specific *allergen.* Because food is produced in a completely allergen-free environment, allergic individuals have the highest level of assurance that this food is safe to eat.

Double-blind test: A *food-allergy* treatment study in which neither the researchers nor the patients know who is receiving treatment and who is not until after the study has been completed.

Eczema: An itchy and persistent red rash characterized by extreme dryness. The condition is commonly referred to as *atopic dermatitis.*

Enzyme: A substance that initiates the body's chemical reactions. *Food intolerances* can be caused by enzymatic defects in the digestive system because the body doesn't have the particular enzyme necessary to digest that food.

Epinephrine: Also known as adrenaline, a hormone, and a neurotransmitter. Increases heart rate, contracts blood vessels, dilates air passages, and participates in the fight-or-flight response of the nervous system. It is available by prescription as EpiPen® or Twinject®, delivered via a shot, and now as Auvi-Q™, a battery-powered compact epinephrine device that talks a user through the injection process step by step. It is your best defense in controlling severe allergy and/or anaphylactic reactions.

False positives: A *food-allergy* skin test result that mistakenly demonstrates that a patient is allergic to a food when he or she is not.

Food allergen: A substance in a food, usually a *protein,* that triggers an allergic overreaction within the *immune system.*

Food allergy: A condition that results when the body's *immune system* mistakenly identifies a particular food as harmful. The body then creates antibodies to that particular food and in turn releases histamine chemicals that cause symptoms of allergic reaction.

Food challenge: Also referred to as the "oral challenge." *Food-allergy* test that consists of a patient consuming the food that he or she is suspected of being allergic to under a qualified doctor's close supervision, in a medical facility, and with emergency medications and equipment readily available.

Food intolerance: A different reaction to food that does not involve the *immune system*. The body's inability to digest a particular food or component of that food due to the lack of the enzyme required to break down the food. Symptoms such as diarrhea, constipation, gas, bloating, and abdominal pain may occur.

Food poisoning: A general term for health problems arising from eating food contaminated by bacteria, viruses, environmental toxins, or toxins present in the food itself. Often causes flulike symptoms or symptoms that mimic *food allergy.*

Gluten: *Protein* in wheat and other grains (including barley, rye, oats) that commonly triggers reactions in those with Celiac disease.

Histamine: A chemical released by the body during an allergic reaction; the cause of many of the symptoms of an allergic reaction.

Hives: Multiple red, raised, itchy bumps that form on the skin, often as the result of an allergic reaction. They can appear anywhere on the body.

IgE antibodies: Immunoglobulin E. One of the antibodies that the *immune system* releases during an overreaction to an allergenic food. *Allergists* use a blood test to determine the presence of IgE in order to diagnose or rule out an allergy to a particular substance.

Immune system: The system that protects your body from diseases and infections. When a person has *food allergies,* the *immune system* identifies one or more foods as harmful.

ImmunoCAP test: CAP-RAST test for the diagnosis of *food allergy.* See *RAST.*

Lactase: *Enzyme* required by the body to break down lactose (milk sugar).

Lecithin: A food emulsifier that contains egg and/or soy.

Life cycle: An assessment of every step of the food-making process from growing to final labeling and packaging. This is required to understand whether or not a food contains allergens.

Open test: A *food-allergy* treatment study in which researchers and patients all know who is receiving treatment and who is not.

Oral allergy syndrome: A reaction restricted to the lips and mouth characterized by itching, sometimes severe, and mild temporary swelling. Most often caused by allergies to fresh fruits and vegetables in people with severe pollen allergies.

Placebo: A substance that has no therapeutic effect but is used as a control in testing new drugs or clinical trials.

Plant sterols: A dietary, plant-based compound popular in lowering blood cholesterol levels. Used as an additive in some prepared foods and some heart-healthy orange juices; contains soybean oil and peanut oil.

Protein: A long chain of amino acids present throughout the body and in food. Foods that cause allergic reactions commonly contain proteins that the immune system mistakenly identifies as dangerous.

RAST: Radio-Allergo-Sorbent Test. A blood test that helps diagnose the presence of *IgE antibodies* in a patient to specific foods. Used by a doctor to identify or rule out particular food allergies.

Skin test: A *food-allergy* test in which suspected *allergens* are injected in small amounts below the top layer of skin to determine whether the body reacts to the substance.

Acknowledgments

This book could not have been written without the unflagging support of my family: my daughter Charlotte Jude Schwartz, my beloved Erik Noonan, and my Dad. I'm indebted to many for their expert eyes and ears, beginning with the complete understanding of living with food allergies provided by my family allergist, Dr. Avraham Giannini, who taught us, with humor, that Mom (me) was "not to blame" and that we would find our way. Thank you Bay Area Allergy Advisory Board, Dr. Michel Jean-Baptiste, Dr. Scott Sicherer and The Consortium of Food Allergy Research (CoFAR), Dr. Lisa Dana, our first Bay Area Allergy Advisory Board Chairman Dr. Gary Ross, Kathleen Anderson Ross, James Andrew and Renee Rose Schwartz and the Schwartz family, the Noonan family, Drew Altizer, Joel Goodrich, Karen and Oliver Caldwell, Moya Stone, Gwen Smith and *Allergic Living* magazine, Massachusetts Department of Education, Damion Matthews, Nancy Gregory, Henry McMillan, Julia Bradsher, Maria Acebal, Gina Clowes, FAAN/Food Allergy Research & Education, Tom & Melanie Staggs, Trish Vega, Claudia Castillo Ross, Elizabeth Landau, Helen Holt and Jonathan Lawhead, Carole Jelen at Waterside Productions, Zachary Romano, Norman Goldfind, Susan E. Davis, and Brian Hom and family.

Special thanks to:

- The Consortium of Food Allergy Research (CoFAR) for permission to reprint "How to Read Labels to Avoid Food Allergens" in Chapter 3 and "Summer Camp and Food Allergies" in Chapter 5.

- Food Allergy Research & Education for permission to reprint in Chapter 5 all its Food Allergy Management in Schools documents, including "Food Allergy School Checklist," and "Suggested Guidelines for Family, Camper, and Camp," and in Chapter 8 its "Food Allergy Valentine Checklist."

- Select Wisely for permission to reprint examples of their international language cards for food-allergic travelers in Chapter 7.

Index

About the Author

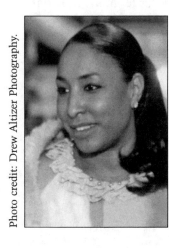

Photo credit: Drew Altizer Photography.

Mireille Schwartz is allergic to fish. She was a member of the Board of Directors for Washington, D.C.-based FAAN (Food Allergy & Anaphylaxis Network; now Food Allergy Research & Education) from 2009 to 2011. FAAN is the world's leading nonprofit allergy resource that works with policymakers on federal, state, and local initiatives in such areas as food labeling, epinephrine availability, and management of food allergies in schools, camps, airlines, and restaurants. In 2009 and 2010, Mireille was named honorary chairman of the San Francisco FAAN Food Allergy Walk-A-Thon, alongside Academy of Country Music award winner and "Celebrity Apprentice" finalist Honorary National Chairman Trace Adkins. In both 2009 and 2010, Mireille was awarded FAAN's National Award of Appreciation.

Mireille Schwartz is CEO and founder of the Bay Area Allergy Advisory Board established in 2007. The board's mission is to promote education, awareness, and provide no-cost medical care and medication to Bay Area families with severely allergic children.

In September 2010, Mireille was honored by Senator Mark Leno with a California State Senate Award for commitment to raising awareness, education, and advocacy on food allergy and anaphylaxis. Mireille also received a 2009 Change Starts at Home Changemaker's Award for outstanding stewardship and advocacy for food-allergic children, and The Huffington Post's "Greatest Person of the Day" Award in July 2011. Additionally, Mireille and her family were featured in the 2013 Discovery Channel documentary "An Emerging Epidemic: Food Allergies in America," narrated by Steve Carell.

An expert contributor to CNN Health, National Public Radio, Yahoo! News, and ABC7 News, and a featured "Adult Allergies" columnist in *Allergic Living* magazine, Mireille has an innate understanding that food is everywhere, and our relationship to food needs to be healthy if we are to stay healthy. Mireille Schwartz lives in San Francisco, California, with her family.